The Hospital

By such means, Dr Mahler concludes, may hospitals 'be converted into agents for the service of society instead of precincts for individual medical transactions between doctors and patients... [and] become one of the main flag bearers of the most promising health movement in the history of humanity...[1].

The Hospital

From centre of excellence to community support

Norman Vetter

Senior Lecturer in Epidemiology and Public Health at the
University of Wales College of Medicine, Cardiff, UK

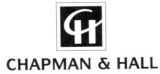

CHAPMAN & HALL

London · Glasgow · Weinheim · New York · Tokyo · Melbourne · Madras

Published by Chapman & Hall, 2–6 Boundary Row, London, SE1 8HN, UK

Chapman & Hall, 2–6 Boundary Row, London SE1 8HN, UK

Blackie Academic & Professional, Wester Cleddens Road, Bishopbriggs, Glasgow G64 2NZ, UK

Chapman & Hall GmbH, Pappelallee 3, 69469 Weinheim, Germany

Chapman & Hall USA, 115 Fifth Avenue, New York NY 10003, USA

Chapman & Hall Japan, ITP-Japan, Kyowa Building, 3F, 2-2-1 Hirakawacho, Chiyoda-ku, Tokyo 102, Japan

Chapman & Hall Australia, 102 Dodds Street, South Melbourne, Victoria 3205, Australia

Chapman & Hall India, R. Seshadri, 32 Second Main Road, CIT East, Madras 600 035, India

Distributed in the USA and Canada by Singular Publishing Group Inc., 4284 41st Street, San Diego, California 92105

First edition 1995

© 1995 Norman Vetter

Typeset in 10/12 Times by Saxon Graphics Ltd, Derby
Printed in Great Britain at Hartnolls Ltd, Bodmin

ISBN 0 412 61060 4   1 56593 417 2 (USA)

A catalogue record for this book is available from the British Library

Library of Congress Catalog Card Number: 94–74683

♾ Printed on permanent acid-free text paper, manufactured in accordance with ANSI/NISO Z39.48-1992 and ANSI/NISO Z39.48-1984 (Permanence of Paper).

Contents

Acknowledgements

I would like to acknowledge the assistance given to me in the preparation of this book by Dr Lise Llewellyn for helpful comments and Ms Julia Evans for her help in wordprocessing it.

Introduction

Hospitals arouse strong emotions. Doctors, nurses and therapists, remembering the excitement of their early training years, associate hospitals with youth, vigour and the possibilities presented by a new career. The heady mixture of large numbers of young men and women exploring new ideas together remains as an affectionate memory with most medical professionals for the rest of their working lives.

For the general public the perception is different. Most people fear the prospect of entering a hospital, even as a visitor. This is, ultimately, because numbers of people who enter hospitals die there. Hospitals have an alien feel for most members of the general public, which is not understood by people who work in them. Friends not working in medicine mention the confusing diversity of uniforms, the bustle to no obvious purpose and the patronizing way that people are treated, as reasons for their dislike.

These are feelings common to any group of outsiders finding themselves in a closed world. Doctors and nurses feel similarly when visiting law courts. Most hospitals, however, give out a feeling of threat that is unique. It is often described in terms of the smell. This threat is so great that hospitals are still used as a threat to pacify small children, especially the threat of being locked up in one of the large mental hospitals. Oddly, and despite this, the one issue which brings people out onto the streets to defend health facilities is the attempt to close a hospital.

NUMBER OF HOSPITALS OVER THE PAST 20 YEARS

Despite their importance to doctors, nurses and the general public, hospitals are disappearing fast and have been doing so for many years. Figure 1.1 shows the number of hospitals in England over the past 20 years [2]. There has been a rapid and constant fall in their numbers over that time amounting to a reduction by one-third since 1970.

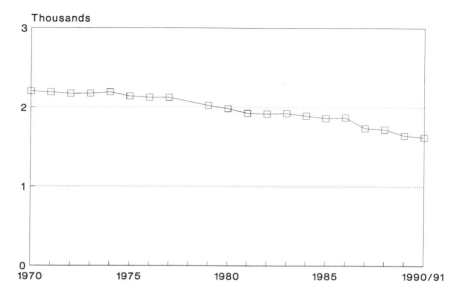

Figure 1.1 Number of hospitals in England.

The reduction in the number of hospitals may not be a reduction in the number of places. It could be that the reduction in the number of hospitals is due to small hospitals closing, and a smaller number of large ones taking their place. To clarify this, Figure 1.2 shows the number of places for patients, usually defined as the number of beds, contained in the hospitals over the same period. There is, if anything, an even more rapid fall in the numbers of beds, the reduction has been fastest in the last 3 or 4 years.

The most dramatic thing about these figures is that they are so consistent. If a line joining the number of beds is extended, it crosses the zero point in the year 2029/2030. This suggests that the last National Health Service (NHS) bed will vanish during that year.

When one looks at the specialties separately, the main fall in the number of beds is in the field of mental illness and in acute medical and surgical beds. There has, in contrast, been a very slight rise in the number of beds in geriatrics, the care of elderly people (Figure 1.3).

This apparently clear cut story is complicated by looking at the number of cases treated in hospital each year. Figure 1.4 shows the data over the same time period as that for beds. This shows a steady increase in the number of cases seen per annum from 5 million in 1970 to 6.5 million in 1987. The numbers are increasing at a steady rate, except in the last 4 years on the graph, where for 2 years there is a levelling off, then a jump, then a levelling once again. The jump,

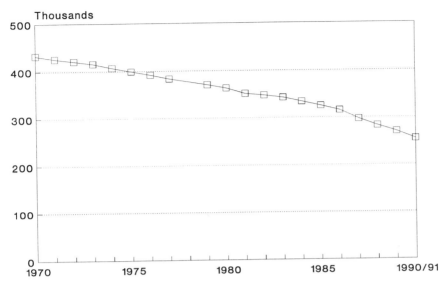

Figure 1.2 Number of hospital beds in England.

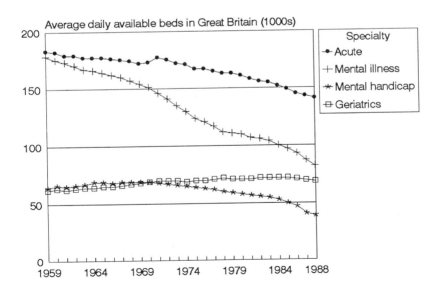

Figure 1.3 Available beds in most specialties have fallen in number except in geriatrics.

in 1986/1987 was due to a change in definition of what constitutes a patient in hospital. Assuming the two levelling off years are artefacts one is left with the odd conclusion that, as the last hospital bed closes in 2030, between 12 and 14 million cases will be seen in that remaining bed during the year.

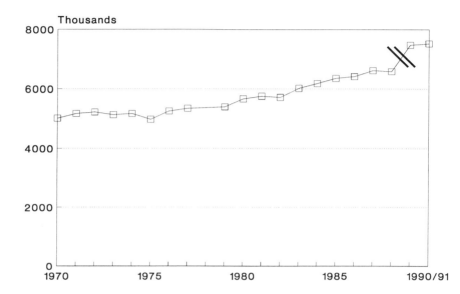

Figure 1.4 Number of cases treated in England.

This conundrum suggests, if nothing else, that the nature and use of hospitals is changing rapidly and will continue to do so in the future. My thesis, in this book, is that the pressures which have caused these changes will continue to increase, so that hospitals, as we recognize them today, will cease to exist. The changes to hospitals will be the most obvious indication to the public of equally extensive changes in the practice of medicine, nursing and the other health professions. Also, if we have the foresight to bring it about, there will be a creative change in the way that people view illness and health.

HISTORICAL DEVELOPMENT OF HOSPITALS

Until the dissolution of the monasteries, institutions for the sick were usually linked with houses run by religious orders. They formed an important part of the spread of Christianity throughout Europe. These religious houses were centres of learning and provided spiritual help for the local community as well as offering safe havens for travellers. Hospitals therefore in their earliest form both provided care for the sick and acted as hotels [3]. They also acted as homes for orphans and others who were unable to maintain themselves.

The people working in these early hospitals had a limited knowledge of the treatment or cure of disease and were therefore mostly confined to keeping people comfortable and ready to meet their maker. The religious community did help to promote practical ideas relating to public health in its own institutions, in the development of toilet blocks, draining systems and provision of clean water. These ideas were slow to catch on in the homes of the population at large, but the ideal was there to be copied by those who could afford it. This is one of the early examples of ideas developed in the institutions being translated for use by the local community.

The closure of the monasteries by Henry VIII and the resulting loss of their medical expertise was a spur to the development of the medical profession, which then developed outside its religious origins. The first sign of this early reorganization of the health services was the foundation of the Royal College of Physicians, which, in 1518, began licensing London doctors.

Thomas More, chancellor under Henry VIII, oversaw considerable improvements in London's general water supply. His friendship with the first president of the Royal College of Physicians, Thomas Linacre, led him to suggest a number of public health measures, which became widely publicized in his famous book, *Utopia*. He also suggested that people infected with the plague should remain in their own homes rather than be taken to an institution because of the dangers of cross infection.

It is interesting that this problem, of whether to move highly infectious individuals into institutions, has remained a difficulty down the ages. It was made apparent to me in Bangladesh in the mid-1970s during the Smallpox Eradication Programme. An important way of reducing the spread of the disease was keeping people in their own homes. In Bangladesh this took the draconian form of two hired guards who had strict instructions not to let the patient leave his or her home, and certainly not to let him or her go to hospital. Hospital care was of no help to patients at a personal level. Food, drink and other comforts were provided by the family wherever the patient was kept and there was no treatment available which could not be given as easily in the home. The danger for the individual patient lay in being wrongly diagnosed as having smallpox, being admitted to the smallpox ward and then contracting the disease. Infected patients were also a grave danger to others in hospital who did not have smallpox, at a time when they were particularly vulnerable from the effects of other diseases.

A number of vicious outbreaks in widely dispersed areas had followed the practice of admitting patients. This was because relatives travelled considerable distances to visit patients who had been admitted, making the possibility of spread to the general population very real. This, of course, presupposes that patients admitted to hospital were not fully isolated from others, as was the case in Bangladesh at that time. The problem was pinpointed further when a hospital employee in Birmingham, in the UK, contracted smallpox from a research laboratory after the last case had been eradicated in Bangladesh. Thomas More appears to have been aware of these dangers more than 400 years ago. It was a salutary lesson for me, being the first time that I had come across the hospital as a cause of, rather than a cure for, disease.

In 1601, parishes became, for the first time, responsible for the care of old and chronically ill poor people and fatherless children. This led to the development of workhouses, some of which had their own infirmary. The well-to-do, with servants to do their nursing, and able to afford a doctor to visit them, were treated in their own homes.

In the 18th century increasing numbers of rich benefactors founded voluntary hospitals, many of which still exist today, often on the original site and occasionally in the original building. They remain the 'better heeled' hospitals and at the time were particular about who they admitted. Figure 1.5 shows the rules of admission to hospital for the Edinburgh Royal Infirmary built at that time, together with a translation of the original entry.

The advance of industrialization during the 19th century led to the rapid growth of cities owing to the lure of work in the towns and the introduction of machinery allowing for less labour intensive methods on the land. The social changes were, as so often seems to be the case, accompanied by a rapid rise in the birth rate, resulting in more babies and children at risk and a rapid increase in poverty in this group. These changes, together with increased travel, within the country on the railways and internationally by ship, led to a downturn in the health of the nation, especially with regard to infectious diseases, as previously isolated individuals and communities were brought into contact with one another.

This, in turn, stimulated an interest in public health, as distinct from individual care. The connection between poor social conditions and poor health became obvious. The elder statesmen of the public health specialty set about campaigning for changes in the law that would help to overcome those social conditions, rather than trying to cure sick individuals. These laws culminated in the Public Health Act of 1875, sometimes called its 'Magna Carta'. This was championed by a prominent physician, Sir John Simon.

The act made compulsory the appointment of a Medical Officer of Health for each local authority and aimed to ensure drainage, refuse removal and the isolation of infected persons. In this instance isolation was to be brought about by the removal of that person to special hospitals. Whether these changes to the external environment were responsible for the gradual subsequent improvement in health, or whether this was due to the increasing wealth of the population and hence their ability to purchase heating, food and clothing is not clear. It was probably a mixture of both. It certainly had little to do with developments in personal medicine or the provision of hospital care [4].

Hospitals expanded and increased in number during the 19th century. Several pressures were responsible for this expansion. One was the presence of rich men who had made their money as industrialization progressed. There was also a

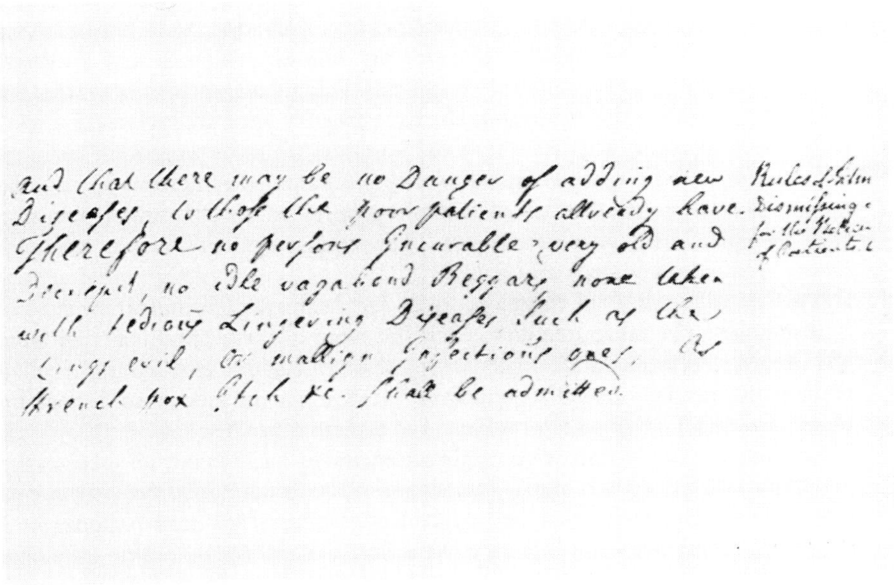
And that there may be no Danger of adding new
Diseases, to those the poor patients allready have.
Therefore no persons Incurable, very old and
Decrepit, no idle vagabond Beggars, none taken
with tedious Lingering Diseases, Such as the
Kings evil, or mallign Infectious ones, As
ffrench pox Itch &c. shall be admitted.

From Infirmary Minute Book, vol. 1. page 37 (2 November 1730)

Rules of Admitting, Dismissing and for the Behaviour of Patients contd.

And that there may be no Danger of adding new Diseases to those the poor patients allready have Therefore no persons Incurable, very old and Decrepit, no idle vagabond Beggars, none taken with tedious Lingering Diseases, Such as the King's evil or mallign Infectious ones, As ffrench pox Itch &c. shall be admitted.

Notes: King's evil = scrofula
Itch = scabies

Figure 1.5 Copy of the Edinburgh Royal Infirmary minute book for 2 November 1730.

growth in civic pride and a feeling of responsibility for 'the public' which resulted in the development of public buildings of all sorts, from hospitals and schools to libraries and public baths. Doctors who were Members of the Royal Colleges dominated the voluntary hospitals, which developed into centres for research and teaching. The consultants gave their services free to treat the sick and poor in hospital, while earning their fees from their work outside the hospital, either in general practice or as private consultants. The rich still opted to be treated at home with the necessary services being brought in, rather than mix with the poor and possibly infectious. The middle classes were increasingly drawn to the new hospitals for treatment.

Medical students paid to study under the hospital consultants, who were regarded as the cream of the profession and were restricted to more traditional specialties, medicine and surgery in particular. As the century wore on a number of doctors founded voluntary hospitals in single specialties, especially for the treatment of eyes and ears, nose and throat.

The voluntary hospitals were originally intended for the poor but because of the prestige of the doctors using them, more people sought to be treated there as outpatients, rather than go to their general practitioners. Workers organizations and friendly societies developed subscription systems so that their members could get free treatment from the voluntary hospitals when they needed it.

This was seen by general practitioners as a threat to their living and caused considerable professional jealousy between the general practitioners and the consultants. This conflict was gradually sorted out by an informal professional agreement, though some would say that the animosity built into the system in those years has remained until the present day. By the late 19th century, hospital doctors with specialist knowledge increasingly acted as consultants for other doctors, including general practitioners, where the case had some aspect of special interest.

Infirmaries and asylums, originally part of the Poor Law institutions, were gradually separated from the workhouses. In time they became available not simply to the indigent poor, but also to the general public under the aegis of the local authorities, the successors to the parish. Doctors working in these hospitals were paid a salary for doing so [5].

Concerns about providing health care, especially to poor people, grew, so that in 1911 David Lloyd George introduced a bill to provide compulsory national insurance for manual workers with incomes below £160 per annum. A contribution of 4d per week by the person insured together with 3d by the employer and 2d from the Government gave them three main benefits: cash for any period of incapacity which made them unable to work; the costs of general practitioner care; and drug costs. The bill was administered by 'approved societies', mainly the friendly societies that had previously provided voluntary insurance. Some insurance companies and trade unions were also approved.

These societies appointed doctors on a 6s a year capitation fee for medical attendance and drugs. The patients had no freedom of choice about which doctor they could see, neither were doctors in any way involved in the administration of the Act. The Act did not affect hospitals, though some central government funds were provided for setting up tuberculosis sanatoriums. The societies administering the Act were, however, authorized to make grants to voluntary hospitals, thus enabling some relatively poor working people to make use of them.

THE NATIONAL INSURANCE ACT

Hospitals feared that the National Insurance Act would cause a massive drop in their subscriptions as patients deserted their outpatient departments for the free service, but this did not come about. It did, however, lead to a reversal of the position of hospitals and general practitioners in the distribution of patients. Hospitals, fearing that they would run out of money, turned away some of the outpatients that they had previously welcomed and treated free of charge because the general practitioners (who were paid according to the number of people on their list, a capitation system) now tended to send their more difficult and time-consuming patients to hospital.

The hospital continued to move towards being a specialist consultation centre, even in its outpatient departments, although general practitioners still did some specialist work in areas that were short of manpower, such as anaesthetics and obstetrics. General practitioners also had some beds for inpatients in their cottage hospitals and nursing homes. The voluntary hospitals continued to suffer from increasing financial pressure and, as a result, introduced charges and a few pay bed wards for middle class patients. Charges consisted of a contribution from patients according to a means test. If local authorities sent patients to the voluntary hospital they would pay the charges if the patients were poor. Voluntary hospital consultant staff continued to be unpaid for their hospital work and to enjoy high status.

The public, local authority-run hospitals were by the 1920s attempting to care for all the patients in their catchment area. They provided three-quarters of the hospital beds, though, because as these patients tended to have chronic diseases and to be elderly, they tended to be in hospital for long periods. As a result, they probably served considerably less than three quarters of the population. The finance for the public hospitals was found mainly from the local councils and grants from central government. Unlike the voluntary hospitals, all of the staff were paid. As well as the chronically ill and elderly people, public hospitals tended to take infectious, maternity and mental cases, while the voluntary hospitals gave acute and short-term care for general medical and surgical patients.

In 1920, the Dawson council suggested the development of preventive and other services around health centres, some to be designated as primary centres, others as secondary. Primary health centres would be run by general practitioners with some assistance from visiting consultants and would deal with the simpler cases. Complicated illnesses would be sent to the secondary health centres staffed by consultants and specialists. The development of such community based health services was to be suggested at regular intervals over the following 70 years. This approach is similar to the one that I believe is likely to develop in the UK over the next 10 years owing to the pressures that I outline later. This will make the large general hospitals redundant. I believe that the time is now ripe for these changes, but Dawson probably thought so too.

Between 1918 and 1939 a number of other committees encouraged ideas for putting the existing two-hospital system on a sounder footing, particularly because of the financial crises regularly facing the voluntary hospitals. Most of the suggested reforms were strongly resisted by the medical profession, because of its fears of state control. A Royal Commission in 1926 first suggested that the only way for the majority of the population to be able to enjoy costly medical services would be to pay for the services through general public funds.

In 1933, the Socialist Medical Association first suggested the provision of a free, tax-supported service on a universal basis with doctors working on full-time salaries and with full professional freedom. The service was to be organized around health centres for outpatient care and large general hospitals for institutional care. The administration was to be looked after by local authorities. This programme was incorporated into the Labour Party programme in 1934.

WORLD WAR II

The demands on hospitals made by casualties during World War II pinpointed the awkward complexity of the system as it stood, especially that of the voluntary hospitals. During the war, voluntary hospitals were well paid for their beds but, despite this, they still tried to reject long-term and elderly patients, supposedly in order to have as many emergency beds available as possible. The Emergency Medical Service, set up for the treatment of war casualties, employed hospital doctors on a full-time salaried basis.

These changes were partial and short-term but they did change public attitudes towards hospital care, so that the need for a large scale reorganization of the existing services was obvious. It has been argued that World War II saved the voluntary hospitals from financial disaster but it also emphasized the great financial problems that they had and led finally to their being integrated with the local authority hospitals.

The Beveridge Commission Report of late 1942 [6] assumed that the health of the nation was poor because of a lack of access to health services. Knowledge of the nation's health, as during World War I, was brought to the attention of the authorities by the large proportion of men who were found to be unfit to join the forces during conscription. The report was not specific on financing but appears to have assumed that a national insurance system would be used.

Beveridge envisaged that regional bodies, based on medical schools, which had been the most prestigious of the voluntary hospitals, would plan services and develop the funds for the region in conjunction with the remaining voluntary hospitals. The local authority hospitals would stay under the care of local authorities, but the two systems would be coordinated by a Medical Advisory Committee.

The voluntary hospitals rejected the idea of a joint authority. They feared that there would not be true partnership between the public and voluntary hospitals and assumed that the regional authorities would favour the public hospitals. It was suggested that the voluntary hospitals should still have to provide some of their own finance. The British Hospitals Association, representing the voluntary hospitals, made the point that it would be difficult for them to attract other finances if a free hospital service also existed.

THE NATIONAL HEALTH SERVICE ACT

The National Health Service Bill, when it was eventually published in 1946, proposed that all the population be covered for all costs and that the health services should be free for all at the time the service was used. The most important change of policy that the bill brought about for hospitals was to nationalize them all and bring them together, administered in regional groups, covering populations of 2–3 million, generally with a medical school at the hub of each. These regional hospital boards administered the planning and development of hospital services.

A second tier of management committees, one for each large hospital or group of smaller hospitals, was responsible for the day-to-day operation of the hospitals. These were appointed by the regional board after consultation with the local authority and the medical and dental staff of the hospitals concerned; the members of these committees were taken mainly from these groups. The health minister and, under him, the regional boards controlled the finances. The teaching hospitals were to have boards of governors, some appointed as for a regional board but also some members to be nominated by the university. These boards were to receive the endowments of the hospital concerned to be used as they wished.

The split was now between teaching and non-teaching hospitals. Local government representatives who, as a result of these changes, had lost their own hospitals, were very critical of the boards on the grounds that the appointees were not democratically elected, though in practice a proportion of the membership of the boards was drawn from elected councillors. The Royal Colleges welcomed the changes, at least partly because of the good level of remuneration for consultants, who would be salaried according to the proportion of their time they gave to the health service. In addition, a distinction award scheme was brought in, which was meant to compensate high prestige consultants for the loss of private income which a commitment to the NHS would entail.

General practitioners were critical. They were paid a capitation fee according to the number of patients they had on their lists, administered by a Family Practitioner Committee. They lost what few rights they had left to manage patients in the voluntary or local authority hospitals, though they retained their cottage hospitals. The non-general practitioner community based services, especially nursing and community medical services, were retained by the local authorities under the direction of the Medical Officer of Health. It was this group that was also responsible for the growing welfare services, later to form full blown social services departments.

This 'tripartite' system of health provision further weakened the contact between general practitioners and hospital consultants and, in turn, primary and secondary care. There was a belief that doctors who passed their finals and did not want to take any more examinations would become general practitioners. Others, said to be the clever ones, would take more postgraduate examinations in order to become specialists and would work in hospital. There was a feeling that general practitioners were therefore second class doctors, condemned to the management of diseases that were common and rarely killed patients and that were therefore of little consequence.

Specialization in the hospitals increased steadily after 1948. The number of Royal Colleges, which controlled the membership of their specialist groups, increased in number, covering obstetrics and gynaecology, psychiatry, paediatrics and pathology. The original medical and surgical colleges developed faculties to assist many of these groups to develop into full colleges. Other groups, such as those for anaesthetists and doctors in occupational and public health remain as faculties of the older and larger colleges. The increase in specialization has been mirrored by the increasing complexity of the examinations needed to enter them. Most recently the Royal College of Surgeons developed a third part to its examination for regulating entrance to the subspecialties, such as neurosurgery and cardiac surgery.

The health service struck problems with costs from its inception. A wage freeze in 1949, brought in to curb inflation, brought considerable financial problems, not least to the staff of the new service. The central concept of a free service was never quite carried through. From the beginning the replacement of dentures and spectacles was charged for if the damage was 'due to carelessness'. It was also possible to pay in order to obtain dentures that were better than those said to be clinically necessary and for amenity beds in hospitals, which were usually in a private, better decorated room than the general ward.

An amending act in 1949, under the Labour government, allowed charges to be made for drugs, although this clause was not utilized until some years later. In the spring of 1951, the Labour government introduced charges that would partly cover the costs of dentures and spectacles but with exemptions for some groups. These were considered necessary because of the rising costs of the health service, due to inflation, the increasing demands of patients and the costs of new advances in medical science [7] – familiar laments.

SUBSEQUENT CHANGES

Ten years later the first of many external management consultants was brought in to help reduce the costs of the health service and to sort out the complexities of the tripartite system. It was the first of a long series of changes to the management structure of the health service driven, it seems, by a belief that it must be possible to organize more cheaply any service spending that much money. Two green papers [7a, 7b] suggested the bringing together of the three different health organizations, with the development of area health authorities as the central focus. These were roughly analogous to counties and their areas contained about half a million people. The regional hospital boards became regional health authorities except in Wales, Scotland and Northern Ireland, where the government offices and the Areas split the regional functions.

The central tenet of that management organization was a belief in consensus or team management. Area and regional health teams, consisting of the officers of the authority (an administrator, finance director, doctor and nurse) were expected to reach a consensus on decision making for the authority. Large areas were divided into districts containing about 150 000 people. McKinsey and Co., the management consultants, set up pilot schemes to test these changes.

At the same time, Sir George Godber, in a series of Cogwheel reports [7c], outlined the structure necessary for doctors (hospital doctors and general practitioners) to be able to influence decision making in the health authorities. The development of area medical committees and the supporting subcommittees would allow every doctor a voice in advising the authority. These changes were emphasized because of the diminished voice that the profession had on the health authorities. The dominance of the medical profession over its own administration began to wane as professional administrators, later managers, took over.

These changes in the health service were brought about in 1974. The increasingly specialist nature of the hospital service had, as a spin off, resulted in the closure of many of the small cottage hospitals and general practitioner maternity units in favour of the large district general hospitals. These district general hospitals now formed the backbone of the areas and districts. The hopes for this new structure were very high. All of the doctors and nurses, with the exception of a tiny number in private practice, were under one authority. The promise of guidance from the medical profession, together with consensus management at the top, suggested a recipe for harmony.

Sadly this was not to be. There was quickly a feeling that the advisory structure was too cumbersome. I remember the same documents being discussed by similar groups of people in one forum after another. Some of the discontent may have been engendered by those consultants who had previously successfully exploited the old system and now had to contend with all doctors having the ear of those in charge. It may have been that consensus meant that everyone had a veto. There was some resentment that nurses, who had had little voice until now, had a seat at the top table. Whatever the reason, talk of restructuring began very soon after the system had settled in.

The changes that occurred during the early 1980s were aimed at streamlining the decision making within district authorities. Firstly, by the removal of one of the tiers, in most places the area tier. This left districts in charge and further enhanced the importance of the district general hospitals. Secondly, general managers were brought in at district and regional level to be responsible for the running of the service, ultimately to the Secretary of State. This removed the consensus approach. The managers were the natural heirs to the regional, area and district administrators and were often the same people.

The next move was the removal of the family practitioner committees from the aegis of the health authorities to become separate authorities, known as the family health services authorities. These had their own board and members and were run by a general manager. This was a period when the importance of strong individual management was considered important. At this point each hospital was run by the district general manager, if there was only one district general hospital, or by a unit general manager if there was more than one.

Those in the latter group were to become very important as the potential leaders of trusts in the later reorganization following the NHS and Community Care Act 1990. They formed the group most in favour of the development of trusts. This is to be expected, the princes become restless waiting for the king to die. If they can all become kings, so much the better. The hospitals continued to dominate but under new management. The development of general management, either by design or accident, moved doctors further away from the centre of power, except for a few who moved into management directly. This was a relatively bloodless battle compared with many previous ones and needs to be examined in a little more detail.

THE DOCTORS

The medical profession had developed by the end of the 19th century into a dual profession, with doctors in the high status voluntary hospitals giving their services free and living off their private practice. The old workhouse infirmaries were staffed by salaried doctors. This division between the 'gentlemen and players' continued for many years in the profession, being responsible for the reluctance on the part of the Royal Colleges to accept geriatrics as a full specialty, for instance.

By the time the NHS was formed the centres of excellence were beginning to move from the voluntary hospitals to the medical schools, though some of these were the same establishments. The search for excellence was spurred on by the rapid development of new and powerful drugs and a rapidly growing body of knowledge which was being nurtured and developed. The spotlight therefore subtly moved from the gentleman to the scientist. The three-piece suit gave way to the white coat as the uniform of a specialist. The stethoscope, instead of being large, cumbersome and 'grey to go with one's grey suit, black to go with one's black suit' (attributed to Sir Derrick Dunlop), moved from being a badge of rank to become a scientific instrument and somewhat smaller.

Doctors who were training to become specialists in the new health service were largely restricted to the teaching hospitals and this is still so. However, the development of specialization for those who had reached the rank of consultant was not confined to the teaching centres. It rapidly became the norm for consultants in district general hospitals, as they developed in the 1960s and 1970s, to move from medicine or surgery into, for instance, cardiology, renal medicine or thoracic surgery.

HOSPITALS AND THE DOMINANCE OF MEDICINE

It should be obvious from the description so far that the medical profession is not a single church. Hospital consultants (especially those in medicine, surgery and their super-specialties, cardiology and neurosurgery) continue to be perceived as the leaders of the profession. Other specialties, notably those that grew up in the workhouse infirmaries – such as the care of elderly people, the mentally ill, and the chronically sick, and public health consultants – are of lower status.

This status is easily measured for the specialists in the profession have their own yardstick known as the distinction award. This was conceived as part of the NHS Act in 1948 during the negotiations between Aneurin Bevan, the Minister of Health and Lord Moran, on behalf of the Royal College of Physicians. Its aim was to compensate consultants for their loss of private income if they agreed to work within the health service.

Distinction awards continue to exist, despite considerable criticism [8] over the years. Figure 1.6 shows the proportion of consultants in each specialty who had distinction awards in 1980 when the system was under particular attack. Figure 1.7 shows the situation at the end of 1992 [9]. The pattern has changed a little, but not much.

The super-specialists are still more highly rewarded than the generalists; those consultant specialties emanating from the voluntary hospitals are more highly rewarded than those coming from the local authorities. General practitioners were not included in the original negotiations.

Hospitals and the expansion of technology

The impetus for the rapid technical expansion of medical care came about in the mid-1940s with the development of antibiotics. These were so effective that for the first time there appeared to be a purely physical answer to disease that did not depend heavily on either defending the patient beforehand, as with vaccination, or relying largely on his or her natural resilience. Cure of mortal disease became regularly possible. In particular, young people could be defended from bacterial invasion as easily as the fit adult. Even for elderly people the power of infectious diseases was greatly modified, though not as dramatically.

The control of infectious diseases in European and North American countries had the effect of revealing the full impact of cancers, cardiovascular disease and

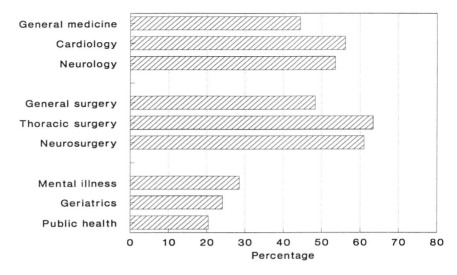

Figure 1.6 Proportion of hospital consultants with distinction awards in 1980.

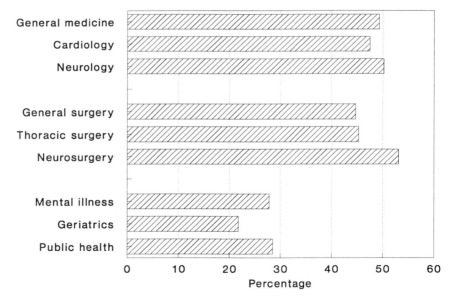

Figure 1.7 Proportion of hospital consultants with distinction awards in 1992.

chronic lung disease as the main causes of death. Their causes are not fully understood, and there is now a consensus that they have no single cause. It is therefore thought to be fruitless to look, except in some rare instances, for some single cause which will, when reversed, cure patients of these diseases. The approaches to treatment have been aimed not at countering the underlying abnormality, but at emergency treatment in the acute phases with removal, in the case of cancer, or replacement in coronary heart disease to reverse the long-term effects.

Attempts to reduce dominance of hospitals

There have been a number of attempts to reduce the power that hospitals exert over the health services, but these have been interpreted as a move to reduce the power of hospital-based specialists and have therefore been greatly resisted. In the 1960s, the so-called 'hospital plan' published by the government at that time [10] suggested the development of large health centres for general practitioners, sometimes on the same premises as the local authority, later known as community health clinics. This was intended to boost the development of the general practitioner-based services. The 'primary health care teams' in these health centres would, it was hoped, develop more preventive services and reduce the pressure on casualty and outpatient departments in district general hospitals.

The enthusiasm for health centres was partly triggered by an enthusiasm for the 'polyclinics' developed in the Eastern bloc countries and some areas of Scandinavia, where the great majority of the health care needed by a local population would be carried out. This could include minor surgery and some specialist outpatient facilities. The hospital plan also suggested the development of the district general hospitals. This part of the plan was taken up with gusto.

The community part of these ideas was undermined by a number of developments. Most important of these was that the district general hospitals took the lion's share of the money available. The system of allocating money, based on a policy which gave everyone what they had last year plus a percentage, was not capable of taking money back from the power bases in the hospitals in large enough quantities to allow innovative ideas to develop. Apart from a few lone voices [11], there was no thought that money should be taken from the 85% of medical interventions for which there is no solid scientific evidence [12].

General practitioners were not allowed to develop community services in many areas. In particular they were discouraged from working alongside the community nurses and local authority clinics where the rest of the community based medical staff were based. This was largely because of the jealousy between the local authority based Medical Officer of Health who ran the community services and the general practitioner services. General practitioners were also somewhat hazy about the work that nurses could carry out in their practice [12a]. The movement towards large health centres petered out. In the last few years, general practitioners who were based in the same premises as the clinics have seen great financial advantages in owning their property, rather than renting it, and have moved out into new premises.

In the 1970s, there was another attempt to divert funds within the hospital service from acute care towards the rehabilitation and long-term care services. At that time, these were largely hospital based, mainly in the former local authority hospitals. This move was partly fuelled by a number of scandals in hospitals for mentally ill, learning disabled and elderly people. The general attitudes of society towards minorities had also changed as evidenced, for example, by the civil rights movement in the USA and the anti-Vietnam war groups. They suggested that, given normal social surroundings, many of the problems these people had would be solved.

These well-meaning moves once again petered out, though a few changes were made, especially the setting up of a number of research facilities. Much of the work of these research groups into the 'normalization' [13] of learning disabled and mentally ill people [14], the development of community care [15], and the problems of elderly disabled people [16] and those who care for them [17], laid the foundations for developing the policy of moving learning disabled and mentally ill people out of long-term hospital care. They also influenced the community care part of the NHS and Community Care Act 1990.

MOVES TO COMMUNITY CARE: MENTAL ILLNESS

The first developments in the services for mentally ill people form a useful framework for showing the sort of difficulties which confront any health service moving from the hospital into community based services. Figure 1.8 shows the changes in the number of inpatient places in England and Wales and in the USA for mentally ill people over 100 years.

It can be seen that the number of places in mental illness hospitals has risen and fallen again over the period in all three countries, but much more dramatically so in the USA. The first widespread schemes to move patients from hospital to community care were in Italy and the USA.

In the UK, the move from hospital based to community based care has been slow. Figure 1.9 shows some basic data on the change in the numbers of places used in hospital and in the community since 1975. It can be seen that there is a considerable shortfall between the places developed and the numbers planned, so that many of the patients discharged from hospital seem to disappear. An important problem with the development of services outside hospital is that it is more difficult to keep track of patients who need follow-up services at regular intervals. The Care in the Community study showed, by studying one area, that the development of services in the community was slower than the rate at which patients were discharged [18]. In addition, there are problems with the degree of priority given to mentally ill people in different places (the cost of health and social services are £17 per person in Wessex RHA compared with £28 in Merseyside RHA).

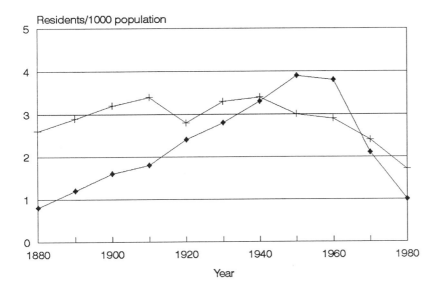

Figure 1.8 Residents in psychiatric hospitals in England and Wales (crosses) and the USA (diamonds). Reproduced with permission from [21].

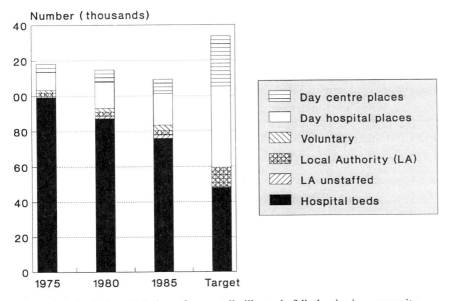

Figure 1.9 As the hospital places for mentally ill people fall, the rise in community places has not kept up.

Nevertheless, successful services have been set up in the UK. In these places, most of the treatment and care is given in the community with back up from acute hospital services. Such an approach has been carried out in Torbay and Derby for some years [19]. In most of the rest of the UK, the plans to follow suit are well advanced. Mentally ill people themselves, with some obvious caveats, prefer community based care. Patients have been shown to become less dependent when given good community services after long periods in hospital. This has been shown to increase their use of shops and pubs, reduce behaviour problems and increase their morale and skills [20].

The mental illness service could therefore be described as a part of the health service that is committed to moving from caring for severely ill people as in-patients towards a service that is based in the area where a patient lives, either delivering services to the home or a small unit close to the home. These changes will make large hospitals unnecessary for mentally ill people. Small local units are likely to be sufficient to cover the need for acute inpatient care.

The changes have uncovered a number of problems which are a pointer to possible trouble for other services moving in the same direction. The reduction in the numbers of mentally ill patients in hospital has been accompanied by very large increases in their use of outpatient services. Unless good, rapid response services are available locally there is a tendency to have a rapid turnover of those patients who do come into hospital. In some areas, a high proportion of the inpatient activities have simply moved from specialist psychiatric to general hospital spending. The result is that the care of mentally ill people, although ostensibly moving into the community, remains largely orientated towards hospital care with nearly 80% of the budget in the UK still going to hospitals. Even in the USA, with its strong commitment to community care, 70% of the spending is on hospital care [21]. It is therefore important not to underestimate the power that hospitals have to hold on to their budgets.

The overall cost of the service seems to have increased. The proportion of gross domestic product (GDP) in the UK spent on mental illness services between 1960 and 1970 remained unchanged but rose by just under one-third between 1970 and 1980 and stayed at a plateau through the 1980s [22]. This was despite the fact that other organizations have been spending more on the mentally ill during that time, on social care and in housing and other services not under the health service budget, for example. The reduction in the health related part of the service has not been reflected in reduced costs [23].

One reason for this is that although the number of residents in hospitals has gone down, only a small proportion of the mental hospitals in the UK have closed completely. The main way in which savings can be brought about in the service are by the closure of large units. In addition, the staff-to-patient ratios are increasing dramatically; for instance, in England the staff-to-patient ratio increased by just over a third between the mid-1970s and mid-1980s [24]. In other words, there is a tendency, as community care is brought in, for hospitals to become more costly and highly staffed for the number of patients they manage.

The good news is that rising inpatient care costs may accelerate the move towards community care as there are a number of alternatives which appear to be at least as cost effective as conventional inpatient care. Some of these show better results at less cost.

The new changes brought in by the NHS and Community Care Act 1990, to be described in detail later, will also have some impact on changing the rate of inpatient care. In particular, NHS Trusts, whether hospital or community services, will have to pay charges for their capital stock of buildings, land and equipment for the first time. This was intended to allow private providers to compete in a reasonably equitable way with services provided by the health trusts. Given the changed attitude towards the costs of buildings it may well be that the move away from inpatient care will be accelerated.

In addition, the health authority purchasers will be able to put pressure on health and social services providers to work more closely together, a considerable stumbling block for the development of community care in the past. Authorities will be able to buy care from either their own health service providers or from the social services as best fits the needs of the population in the area. This again will increase the opportunities for people to be treated in the community rather than at home.

2

Pressures for change: demographic

AGEING AND THE USE OF HOSPITALS

The main problems faced by hospital services are their increasing costs or the changes needed to make them more efficient. This always seems to come back to the cost of caring for and treating elderly people and the 'burden' that such treatment imposes on the hospital services. There is a feeling that the combination of increasing demands from elderly people and increasing severity of their disabilities will require more and more hospital services and that little of this can be substituted for by services in the patients' homes. This debate about the increasing numbers of elderly people and their potential effect on the health and social services is often led by eminent people, both in the specialized [25] and not so specialized [26] press. Curiously, despite an intuitive feeling that more old people must mean more disabled people and that, in turn, this will lead to more elderly people in hospital, the three components (an ageing society, dependency and the use of health services, including hospitals) are not inextricably linked.

It is true that, as far as hospitals are concerned, quite a high proportion of the hospital beds for the acute specialties, such as general medicine and general surgery, are occupied by people aged 65 and over. Figure 2.1 shows the percentage over the past 20 years in England. It can be seen that the proportion, especially of those over 75, has been increasing gradually, but not dramatically, over that time. There was a change in the way the numbers were collected in 1986/7 accounting for the fall between 1985 and 1987.

These changes may be thought to be relatively unsensational given that the proportion of people aged 75 and over increased in the UK during that time by 50% so that they account for more of the population in real terms and form a greater proportion.

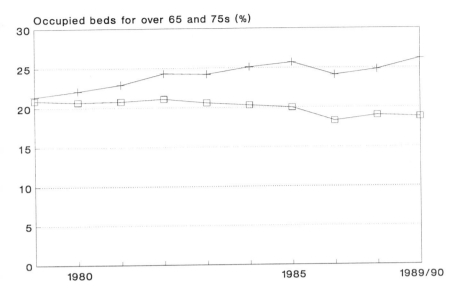

Figure 2.1 The proportion of acute beds occupied by 65–74 year olds (squares) and those over 75 years old (crosses) in England.

Numbers of elderly people in hospital

It is not surprising that the age of hospital inpatients is increasing. Young people are becoming progressively fitter and when they do become ill are increasingly being treated at home. The increased proportion of elderly people in hospital is therefore, to some extent, a reflection of less demand from young people. The small relative increase in Figure 2.1 must give some pause for thought about whether an increase in the use of hospital facilities as a result of the increased age of the population is inevitable. To clarify this we need to examine why there are more elderly people now than in the past.

THE AGEING POPULATION

The population structure of the UK has changed dramatically over the past 150 years. The structure in 1981 is shown in Figure 2.2. The numbers for the UK are compared with those for Malawi which are thought to be similar in shape to those found in the UK about 150 years ago.

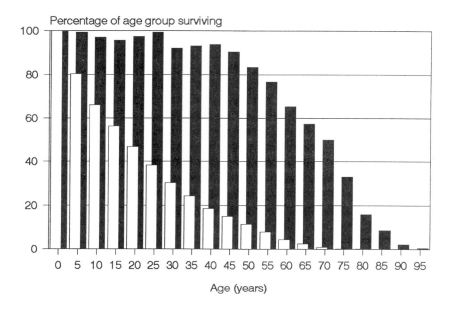

Figure 2.2 Population structure of the UK (unshaded) in 1981 and Malawi (shaded) in 1977, showing the percentage of the population that live to a given age.

The shape of the population profile is markedly different in the two countries. The profiles, typical of those found in developed and developing countries, show the percentage of the population surviving in each age group. In Malawi, the numbers fall rapidly for people aged 0–40 years, then level out for older ages. This curve shows that people of all ages are at quite a high risk of dying and that this likelihood of death is much the same for the young and the old. The reason for this is that the environment is hostile, so that there is a high and constant death rate at all ages.

Some of these hostile environmental factors are external – due to the high prevalence of bacteria and viruses causing infectious diseases and the virulence of these diseases. Others are internal: the population has poor resistance to these diseases because of poor housing, nutrition and sanitation. The two are closely interwoven. The relatively high mortality of people from developed countries who move to or visit developing countries suggests that the external environment also has some effect.

On the other hand, Figure 2.2 shows that people living in the UK have little risk of dying until well into their 60s. This more rectangular shaped curve shows that where the environment is reasonably well controlled because of the wealth available to the general population, deaths occur within a more limited segment of the life span compared. If only a small segment of the age range dies it follows that this will be reflected by the groups who become ill and are admitted to hospital. The converse is that relatively few younger people need to be admitted to hospital. The change towards a late but rapid onset of death is characteristic of countries which have an ageing population.

An increase in the proportion of elderly people is not simply restricted to developed countries. Figure 2.3 compares the situation in Europe and the USA with developing countries. It shows the number of those aged 75 and over in 1985 and the number estimated for 2025 for some OECD (Organization for Economic Cooperation and Development) countries and contrasts this with data for China and India.

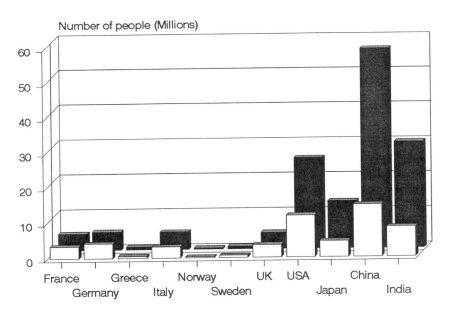

Figure 2.3 International comparisons of the number of people aged 75 and over in 1985 and estimated for 2025.

It can be seen that in the countries shown in the figure both overall numbers and proportional changes in Europe and the USA are overshadowed by expected changes in the principal developing countries, China and India. Within Europe some countries can expect a more rapid rise in the proportion of the population over 75 years old than others. The UK shows fairly moderate changes.

The increase in elderly people

I have mentioned the difference in the environment between developing and developed countries as a factor in the low early death rates in the latter. This is a simplification of the story for European countries. The environment and the resistance of the population to disease has not been as adverse in Europe as in Malawi for many years, yet still there continues to be an increase in the proportion of elderly people admitted to hospital.

The increase in the numbers admitted has been exaggerated by a temporary relative increase in the number of people aged over 75 in the population compared with those between 65 and 74. This was caused by changes in the birth rate of those now aged over 75. Figure 2.4, taken from census data for 1991, shows the number of people alive in the UK in 1991 by age. The graph also shows the number of people born in the corresponding birth year, known as the birth cohort.

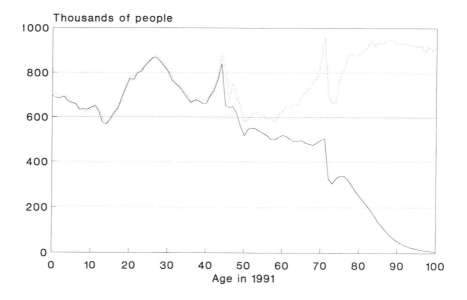

Figure 2.4 The number of people surviving into old age is affected by the number of births. Original births (dotted line); still living in 1991 (solid line).

The curve depicting the number of people alive shows a generally similar outline to that for the UK in Figure 2.3, though there are greater fluctuations in Figure 2.4 because it shows each year separately, whereas Figure 2.3 is smoothed out because the numbers are in 5-year bands. Figure 2.4 shows that the number of births was high when those now between 75 and 100 years of age were born, from the 1890s until 1914. World War I caused a rapid drop in births and this was followed by a post-war rise, reflected in those aged about 70 in 1991. After this births fell markedly during the 1920s.

When those aged 60–70 in 1991 were born, there was a marked fall in the birth rate, whereas in the older groups the birth rate was high. The birth rate fell after World War I as a result of the economic depression in the 1920s. It can be seen that the consequence of the fall in the birth rate in the 1920s was a greater relative number of people aged 75–80 in 1991 than in successive years. The number of people in the birth cohort which was aged 75–80 in 1991 was further exaggerated by reductions in the deaths of infants and young children at that time. These changes were not directly due to medical interventions, but appear to be a response to measures to improve the environment. These changes have been well described and appear to pre-date the important therapeutic advances made by antimicrobial drugs in the 1940s and 1950s [4].

Features of ageing populations

There are a variety of puzzles about ageing in populations and these are likely to have an effect on the extent to which elderly people will need or use hospitals in future. One of the most curious is the difference between men and women. In developed countries and some developing countries the majority of elderly people are female. Figure 2.5 shows the proportion of 80-year-olds who are women in a number of different countries [27].

In general, poorer countries have proportions nearer to 50% than richer, but the pattern is not completely clear. China and Japan, for instance, appear not to fit into this pattern, for Japan is a much richer country than China, with a long lived population, yet is nearer to equality than relatively poor China. The high proportion of women in the older age groups in the UK is reflected in the large proportion of females who need, for instance, treatment for fractured femurs or stroke, and who, as a consequence, form a large part of the hospital population at any one time. It also explains the unequal distribution of elderly women who have no one to care for them, in contrast to the number of elderly men, who usually have a wife still living to care for them.

Those countries where the lifespan has increased, have generally slowed down and often reduced their total population by reducing their birth rate at the same time. This reduction in birth rate means that the other group of dependent people, children, have often shown a decrease in numbers in line with the increase in the numbers of elderly people. This underlines the shift of emphasis in the proportion of people who are dependent on others from the young to the old.

The overall demands of the population on their families do not therefore increase automatically in line with increases in the numbers of elderly people. In fact the general rule seems to be that an increase in the numbers of elderly

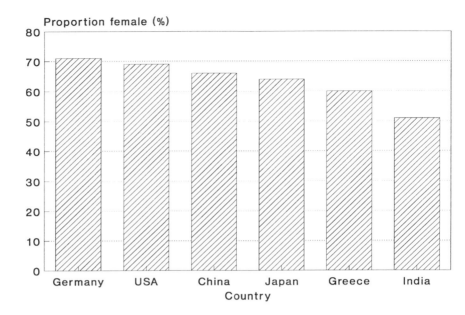

Figure 2.5 The proportion of 80-year-olds who are women. In most countries elderly women form the major part of the elderly population.

people usually accompanies a greater decrease in the numbers of children. Figure 2.6 illustrates this with some more detailed data collected by Benjamin [28]. This shows that as the proportion of elderly people dependent on others has increased, so a number of other groups who are financially dependent have been reduced. The group for which Benjamin found most difficulty estimating future numbers and which appears to have a high level of disability [29] as well as financial dependency, was the unemployed.

It is easier to plan for increases in the numbers of elderly people than fluctuations in the birth rate, or unemployment rate, for there is considerably more warning. Certainly more than 9 months. Children, although dependent on their families for support, are relatively low users of hospital facilities compared with elderly people. Little work has been done on the hospital demands of unemployed people.

The process of ageing and its effect on the disability of the ageing population is complex and the means available to explore such changes are not well developed. Part of the reason for this is the cost of studying changes with time. Researchers need to be young when they start, or they will not see the fruits of their investigations. Despite this, such studies are essential if one of the most important questions about the need for hospital care is to be answered: whether

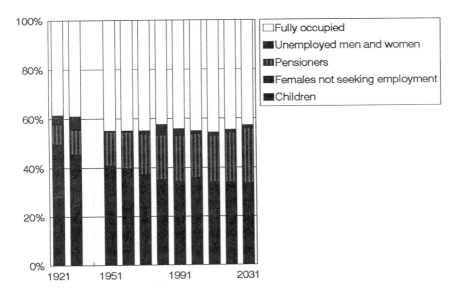

Figure 2.6 The dependent groups in the population over time (with future estimates). (Reproduced with permission from [28].)

countries with increasing numbers of old people also inevitably have an unprecedented need for hospital beds?

The answer to the question involves two subquestions. The first of these is to ask whether having more elderly people in the country automatically means that we will also have more ill people. The second question is whether ill elderly people will be treated in future, for preference, in hospital.

Will more elderly people mean more ill people?

It is often suggested that the present unprecedented increases in lifespan in developed countries will lead to a growth in the proportion of the chronically ill and economically inactive people, therefore causing acute economic problems in the countries affected [26, 30, 31]. Until recently, as I have mentioned, the increase in the proportion of elderly people has not been brought about by people living longer, but by a reduction in the birth rate after World War I [32].

Initially the improved survival of youngsters at that time actually slowed down the ageing of the population. Some of the increase in the numbers of elderly people in the last 10 years is due to middle aged and old people living longer, but there is still no good evidence that this will increase the proportion of disabled people in the community. If people are living longer it seems likely that they are fitter. If they are fitter they may have fewer disabilities. In turn, the proportion of ill and helpless elderly people might even decrease.

I have mentioned that these ideas are difficult to verify or overturn, partly because some people have assumed the answer, and partly because of the difficulty of getting research funding for long-term work. There is some evidence from Sweden that 70-year-old people today are fitter than 70-year-old people were 5 years ago [33]. Cardiovascular risk factors also seem to be reducing with time, presumably improving the longevity of future generations of elderly people [34].

More direct studies have looked at the concept of healthy life expectancy or life expectancy without disability [35]. Using these ideas to study populations of elderly people over time, researchers in the USA have shown that 85-year-old people in 1989 required considerably less assistance to go about their normal lives than they did in 1982 [36]. These researchers also found that community based programmes for caring for elderly people over the long term had greater benefits for both the elderly people and their families, though they were more expensive than hospital based approaches.

One of the few pieces of work carried out on the subject in the UK [37] shows that from 1976 to 1985 there was an increase in life expectancy for both men and women aged 65 and 75. However, when the life expectancy was divided into periods with and without disability (Figure 2.7), the period without disability was seen to increase, whereas the period with disability remained relatively constant, except in the case of women aged 75 who showed no constant trend, rising at first to 1981, then falling again.

There is a another commonly held belief about ageing that is relevant to any discussion about the ageing process and its likely impact on the health services: that humans have a lifespan limit beyond which survival is impossible [38]. As evidence, people quote the fact that members of a single species have similar lifespans compared with members of other species and that the longest lived human was 120 years old [39], which to many people seems low. This suggests that there may be a specific mechanism limiting the lifespan.

However, I have mentioned that, until fairly recently in evolutionary terms, the UK had a similar population profile to Malawi. It can be seen from Figure 2.2 that a tiny proportion of people in Malawi live past reproductive age, so there is no chance of a specific mechanism to destroy people who reached their 70s being developed by evolutionary pressure. There is a growing body of expert opinion which suggests that the limit to human life is simply an accident of history and statistics. There may be no predetermined limit on lifespan and if enough people were born there would be a reasonable chance of one living for ever [32]! The chances are very small.

There is known to be a marked variation in the lifespan of individuals in a group, even in laboratory animals where the environment is virtually identical for all the animals. It is difficult to decide why some individuals live longer than

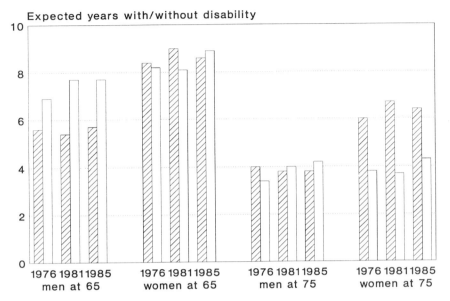

Figure 2.7 Expected years of life without disability (unshaded) rises over time; years with disability (shaded) remain constant. (Reprinted from *Social Science and Medicine,* 27, A.C. Bebbington, copyright 1988, pp. 321–6, with kind permission from Elsevier Science Ltd, The Boulevard, Langford Lane, Kidlington, OX5 1GB, UK.)

others. It does not even have to be a biological phenomenon. An identical collection of atoms of a radioactive substance will not all decay at once, they will produce a 'population decay curve', which looks quite similar to the mortality curves for humans in developed countries [40]. The mortality curve for elderly people at present does not suggest that any form of intervention has had any effect on its shape. In particular, there is no evidence that medical intervention has had any impact.

Causes of death

I have mentioned that in developed countries there is a relatively short period during which people are most likely to die. The possibilities for intervention and therefore prolonging life can be looked at by studying the causes of death. Most of the common diseases in developed countries, such as heart disease, cancers and stroke, rapidly increase in likelihood during the later stages of life. As these different diseases behave similarly to each other the likelihood of suffering more than one also increases with age.

Gavrilov and Gavrilova [33] have suggested that the reason for this is that all organisms, including humans, have a lot of faults that are likely to develop, but a lot of back-up mechanisms for keeping them going when one function fails. It is known that people can survive if they have only about 15% of their liver still functioning or if they have less than one kidney or less than one lung. Quite large quantities of the brain appear to be superfluous. The biochemical systems which keep us going are not especially reliable. There is therefore always a possibility that failure in different parts will coincide and that the person will then be highly vulnerable to any form of illness; the actual diagnosis then becomes irrelevant.

The idea of poor reliability with multiple back-up systems for living things [41], fits in with what is known about the way that many organs work and the shape of the survival curve. Perhaps the most interesting evidence of overabundance of back up is in the genetic structure of the body where the great majority of genes appear to have no useful function. It may be that the working of the evolutionary process requires, or has simply left behind, great quantities of unnecessary material.

An example is found in the genetic basis of some cancers. This suggests that genes may become defective and lead to some types of cancer development. But it appears that several genes at any one time need to become defective for cancer to develop. Defects of a small number of genes may produce harmless tumours, such as warts or cysts, but if more defects form, the tissue may become cancerous.

Once multiple defects occur, whether in genetic material or in other parts of the tissues, almost any disease may cause death. It may be difficult to decide which was the final cause of death. There is a tendency, partly because it requires the chance coincidence of a number of errors, which will itself take time, and partly because some of those errors occur and remain as a cumulative process, for this stage to become more common with increasing age. This state of 'non-specific vulnerability' resulting in a cascade of changes leading to death has been described as 'having one foot in the grave'.

This has important implications for medical practice. A patient in this situation is extremely unlikely to live longer as a result of high tech intervention in hospital. The quality of life of that person will certainly not be improved during the procedures aimed at doing so. The problem reverts from being a technical one of 'how much can we do?' to an ethical one of 'when should we stop trying?'. This decision is about the greater good of a single patient. The more difficult question of when the amount spent on one patient is to the detriment of others will come later.

In a number of international comparisons between causes of death it has been found that there was 'competition' for mortality between different diseases. For instance, stomach cancer and breast cancer in women showed a close relationship, as one increased the other decreased. The same held for breast cancer and tuberculosis. Similar interactions meant that there was little relationship between single causes of death and mortality from all causes. For instance, the contribution of death from cirrhosis of the liver to total mortality is completely compensated for by the effect of other causes of death. Thus if any one cause of death is reduced, it is possible, at least for some causes, that it will have little or no effect on all deaths [32].

For a few diseases the opposite is true. This means that elimination of that disease might save more lives than simply those due to the disease. In the case of early deaths from bronchitis, emphysema and asthma, the relationship between them means that a reduction of deaths due to one would lead to eight times the reduction in overall deaths. It appears that the fight against some types of disease in old people is more effective at reducing total mortality than the fight against others. Such a hypothesis has been suggested to explain the failure of the prevention of coronary heart disease. Lowering the serum cholesterol in a large group of patients reduced the number of deaths due to coronary heart disease, but did not affect the overall death rate [42].

The prospects for prolonging human life are linked not to the elimination of so called premature death, usually defined as deaths in people under 65 years, but to the more practical task of gradually reducing the risk at each age, of being non-specifically vulnerable, which, although less common in younger people, can occur at any age. If this is true it suggests that prolonging human life cannot be greatly influenced by fighting against individual causes of death, single diseases. The stage to tackle is that of preventing vulnerability. There is a corollary to the idea of reaching non-specific vulnerability, mostly, but not always, in old age. That is that many elderly people who are ill have not reached such a state. They therefore respond as well as younger people to medicines which, until recently, were reserved for younger people. Ageism *per se* in the use of powerful treatment will not solve the problems. The right questions to ask concern the overall vulnerability of that person.

In the UK in particular, people aged 70 and over have been discriminated against on the grounds of age alone when decisions have been made about entry to coronary care units and renal dialysis units for kidney failure [43], despite evidence that most complex interventions in screened elderly people are as effective as in younger people. This is the case for coronary artery bypass grafting [44], coronary care [45] and intensive care more generally [46].

Peter Laslett, among others, has made a strong plea for us to try to be more flexible when discussing age. In particular he has suggested the concepts of the third and fourth age [47]. The third age represents the majority of older people who are reasonably fit and who, in medical terms, require to be treated as middle aged people. The fourth age requires a different medical approach. The essential thing to remember is that the difference between the third and fourth age, or indeed between either of them and any other age, is not a matter of chronology. There is no age at which one automatically becomes the other. Perhaps the term third and fourth **age** is a misnomer.

This is relevant to all health care, though at the present time, when the only group being increasingly admitted to hospital is elderly people, these ideas are particularly important for assessing the needs of elderly people for such care. The prevention of vulnerability during the third age, which is the key to improving longevity, needs to be undertaken before people reach that stage, either while they are well or during the attack of a single acute disease. Examples of this protective approach are not fully understood, but cessation of smoking appears to be one important multi-organ protective approach. Some health promotionists have suggested that physical fitness is also important for protecting certain basic reflex mechanisms [48]. There is increasing evidence that countries with the best life expectancy are those that have the most equality between the rich and poor [49]. It is likely to be in this non-specific approach that further improvements to the health of older people lie.

The non-specific vulnerability hypothesis suggests that the rectangular mortality curve seen in the UK is likely to become a little (but not much) more rectangular. It has been shown [25] that, at the moment, in the oldest age groups the curve is flattening out slightly with time. These ideas fit into the observation that there is no age at which the diseases commonly associated with old age suddenly become more prevalent. Death appears as the result of wear and tear phenomena due to a build up of several problems at once, using up all of the large number of back-up systems. This large number of defects is part of what makes each person an individual. We all have a unique set of defects.

SOCIAL ADMISSIONS: NON-SPECIFIC VULNERABILITY?

A group of patients who appear to show characteristics very similar to that called non-specific vulnerability or being in the fourth age has been described [50]. These were elderly patients admitted to hospital with a diagnosis described as 'social and other reasons'. This seemed at first sight to be a non-diagnosis, a rag bag of individuals not easily classified. To our surprise this proved not to be the case.

In the survey of just over 2500 patients aged 65 and over admitted to hospital in Wales, just over 100 patients had a diagnosis of 'social admission' as recorded on their discharge form. They were sent a questionnaire to find out how they had progressed during their stay in hospital. Even before being admitted to hospital those in this group were much more ill than those with other diagnoses. Figure 2.8 shows the large proportion who were severely disabled. Almost two-thirds of the group were housebound compared with less than a quarter of the group as a whole. Incontinence and sensory impairment were about three times commoner in this group than for other admissions. Once in hospital it was found that multiple pathologies were common, with an average of three and a half separate diagnoses per person.

The number of deaths in the first 3 months after leaving hospital were very high. Just over a third of the patients died, compared with about a tenth for other patients of the same age. The main causes of their deaths were heart and circulatory disease, lung disease and cancer. The causes were very similar to those for the rest of the group, simply more common in occurrence and often multiple.

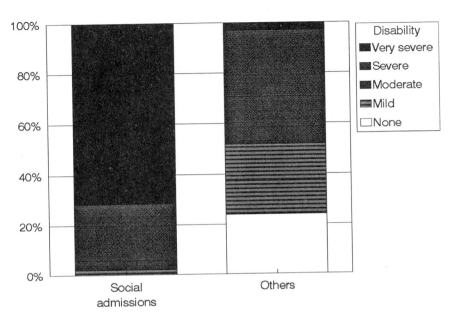

Figure 2.8 Those with social admissions were more severely disabled than others.

The change in severity of disability of people in this group three months after being admitted to hospital was compared with changes in patients with other diagnoses. Figure 2.9 shows that for most patients there was little change in their degree of disability after leaving compared with before entering hospital. The main group, who were not social admissions, appear to be getting worse, but three-quarters of those admitted for social reasons were already severely disabled so they could not be classified as worse, they were already in the worst category. It appears that these patients, if they survive, are not likely to be improved by admission to hospital.

An alternative service to hospital admission could provide the social and nursing care that such patients need. Establishing a national service to provide maintenance and respite care in an environment such as the patient's own home or in nursing homes, seems to be more appropriate than admission to an acute medical or geriatric ward.

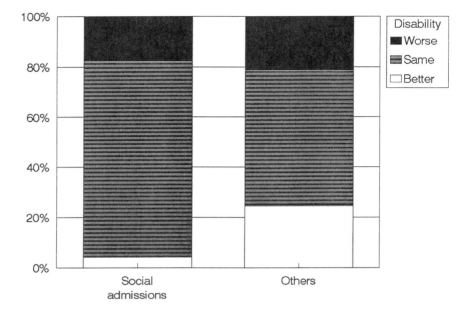

Figure 2.9 Social admissions are not improved by hospital.

WHO SHOULD BE TREATED IN HOSPITAL?

In principle it seems reasonable to avoid admission to hospital whenever possible for all age groups. As far back as 1959, the Platt Committee [51] recommended the extension of community nursing services so that the hospital admission of young children, the other most vulnerable group in society, could be avoided wherever possible. There was little obvious response to this recommendation at the time. The treatment of children in hospital, especially visiting rights for parents, continued to be rudimentary. The Court Report [52], 17 years later, reemphasized the need to avoid admission to hospital, mainly by strengthening the community paediatric services.

Its early recommendations were not taken up, especially the development of general practitioner paediatricians who were to be unusual in the UK as primary care workers, that is professionals with a specialty interest in children to whom people could come directly. Despite this, the stage was set for the expansion of secondary care in the community. Following this report, consultants in community paediatric medicine became increasingly common. From the 1950s until 1980 a few areas paved the way, showing that paediatric care could be provided largely at home, but this did not start to expand rapidly until the 1980s [53].

Should elderly people be treated in hospital?

It is interesting to compare the reasons given for these developments for children with the need for such developments for retired people. The reasons given in the Court Report for extending paediatric home care are to:

- reduce psychological trauma
- prevent cross-infection
- reduce pressure on inpatient beds
- reduce waiting lists
- expand day surgery
- avoid outpatients
- reduce travelling costs
- give more direct support to carers

These reasons seem as valid for elderly people as for young ones. The psychological trauma of moving an elderly person into hospital can result in confusion, delirium and sedation, with loss of control of bladder, bowels and mobility. Cross-infection with increasingly resistant bacteria is a significant problem on wards for elderly people. Inpatient beds for elderly people are constantly under pressure, so that the main indication for discharge in many units is the need for the bed. Waiting lists for some problems of the elderly are difficult to reduce, as the main waiting lists are for surgical treatment. The increasing use of day care may help to alleviate this.

Avoiding admission to hospital is also of benefit to elderly people in less obvious ways. It allows more direct support to carers. It is often assumed that admitting elderly people to hospital alleviates the work of family and friends who may be caring for them and that it is therefore a good thing. This assumption is not borne out by questioning families themselves, who in a number of studies have mentioned the difficulties of visiting elderly people in hospital, especially over a long time. More details will be given on this in the chapters on acute and long-term care.

The hospital care of elderly people therefore appears, for people in the fourth age, to be attempting to concentrate more therapy into a shorter remaining lifespan, where little effect is possible. Often this results in a dreadful final few weeks for extremely frail people. I propose that there are two approaches which can alleviate this part of the law of diminishing returns. First, to concentrate on postponing being non-specifically vulnerable for as long as possible. When it is recognized as existing, we must strive to maintain the elderly person's dignity and quality of life as a higher priority than simply prolonging his or her life. Second, to recognize that people in the third age can benefit from the same acute care as younger people, but that, apart from intensive care, this can be given in the home. Such an approach can lead more naturally to a concentration on improving elderly people's ability to maintain themselves rather than taking over their lives for them.

Do hospitals work for non-vulnerable older people?

A Scottish report on medical rehabilitation stated in 1972 [54] '... at a time when there is an abundance of research on every aspect of the curative, preventive and operational aspects of medicine, there is a striking absence of activity directed towards the benefit obtained from hospital care in its broadest sense, as depicted by the capacity of patients to live an independent and satisfying life after discharge from hospital'.

This is still as true today as it was then. The problem is, if anything, compounded by the increase in the number of dramatic procedures and invasive investigations which are possible, many of dubious effectiveness but certain discomfort. Some of the medical advances of the past 20 years have meant that general practitioners and community nurses can manage much of the work that hospitals have previously had to perform. Medical treatment has taken the place of surgical treatment and has in turn become an outpatient procedure and then a routine task for general practitioners. A good example is the treatment of peptic ulcer, which in the 1960s made up a high proportion of a general surgeon's list, but which can now be treated with medicines given by general practitioners.

One reason that a general overview of the effectiveness of hospitals has been ignored is the difficulty in deciding whether a patient is better as a result of treatment or not. In younger people there has been a tradition of measuring success by whether the patient goes back to work, but this is not relevant to the majority of elderly people. An obvious approach, which seems to have been largely ignored, is to ask the patient if he or she feels better. This is often regarded by doctors and others providing therapy as an outlandish abrogation of responsibility, far too subjective. The attitude seems to be that a patient may be completely cured, but feel awful, or may be still diseased, but feel completely well. The objective truth about the presence or absence of diseased tissue has tended to dominate our measures of the effectiveness of treatments, rather than whether there are still symptoms or whether the patient can carry out the things that are important to him or her.

Another 1972 report on rehabilitation, also largely ignored, summed up the approach [55]: 'The main objective of rehabilitation is to enable the individual to attain the greatest degree of restoration of function, both physical and mental, and if possible, to regain the ability to live independently'.

MEASURING THE EFFECT OF HOSPITAL

A follow-up to the study mentioned above, of over 2500 patients aged 65 years and over admitted to NHS hospitals in Wales [50], looked at discharge preparations [56]. It also showed that one-fifth of all patients died during the year following their admission to hospital. Not surprisingly this was highest in the over 85s where a third died in the year. The highest death rates were among those originally treated for cancers, stroke, coronary heart disease and those admitted for social reasons. About three-quarters of those who died in the year following their admission died of the same thing they went into hospital with. The most common causes of death were circulatory disease, cancer and respiratory diseases.

The patient's disability after discharge was measured using a standard system [57]. Using this measure, one-fifth of patients were worse compared with their state before admission and one in 20 had improved. Two-thirds were no different. A year after leaving hospital a third were more disabled than when they went into hospital, a fifth were less disabled, just under a half were unchanged.

Curiously, older patients did not fare any worse, in terms of their disability rates, than younger patients. It appears that older people are no more likely to be disabled after an acute attack of disease than younger people, if they survive. This appears to be related to the non-specific vulnerability phenomenon. If someone has an illness serious enough to send them to hospital the older ones have a greater chance of dying from it, but if not, their likelihood of being disabled is the same no matter what their age.

Changes in disability were related to patients' diagnoses. Three months after leaving hospital patients who had arthritis, who were admitted mainly for hip replacements, showed the greatest improvement in disability, while stroke patients and those with fractured hips showed the most marked deterioration. Patients with cancer and ischaemic heart disease occupied an intermediate position between these two extremes.

A year after going into hospital, patients admitted originally with a stroke continued to deteriorate, while patients with coronary heart disease showed, on average, a modest improvement in disability. Patients treated for surgical repairs, such as cataract operations or hernia repairs, showed few changes in disability after discharge, but they were, by and large, a fit group of people before they started treatment.

The patients were asked to say what they thought was the effect of their hospital treatment, with the question: 'After your stay in hospital did your health improve, get worse or stay the same?' One year later four out of 10 said that it had improved. Younger patients were more likely to report that treatment had improved their health. Patients with diabetes, prostate disorders, anaemia or bronchitis were the most likely to report improvements to their health as a result of treatment. Least likely to report improvements were patients treated for strokes, fractures or those admitted for 'social reasons', the group mentioned earlier in the chapter.

A substantial fraction of patients were more disabled after discharge than before admission to hospital. The overall impression given of the effect of hospital on disability for these patients was that short-term elective stays, which are increasingly being given as day care, improved people's disability levels, but acute illnesses, requiring emergency admission, were disabling and the hospital stay made little impact on that degree of disability.

Similar results were reported some years ago for younger people in a classic hospital study [58]. The proportion of patients with increasing disability continued to increase after discharge from hospital. Patients' own ratings of their health also became less optimistic as time after discharge increased. This may simply reflect the continuing progression of the chronic disease which underlay the need for acute admission to hospital in the majority of patients. If this is true it suggests that hospital treatment does not appear to have a great deal of effect on the natural history of the commonest diseases now needing hospital admission. Simple acute diseases which are treated and result in complete cure are in the domain of general practice.

Hospital may be worse than useless; it may do harm. Several studies, notably Garraway et al.'s [59] follow-up of stroke patients treated in hospital, have suggested that the loss of the routine of the ward, combined with an overprotective attitude by relatives and carers, may well lead to an increase in disability after discharge from hospital as a direct result of the hospital stay. This may be a more important effect for patients treated in intensive care, for it has been suggested that relatives are more frightened of a condition when the patient gets home if he or she has been treated in a special unit. As a result they tend to inhibit the patient's rehabilitation, for fear of a recurrence of the acute episode. This tendency is increasingly being overcome by complicated regimes to ensure the rehabilitation of patients. The need for psychological support has been known for years in the rehabilitation of patients who have had heart attacks [60], who need considerable psychological help to recover fully [61]. The adverse effects of hospital care are explored in more detail later.

Overall, hospitals in general do not appear to be greatly effective for the treatment of people with chronic disease, mainly older people. The deaths and disability suffered by patients in hospital in the studies mentioned were heavily dependent on the age of patients, their initial disability and their medical condition. These are things which it is not possible to change by treatment in hospital or elsewhere.

Restricting services for elderly people

The cost of health care for elderly people has been a concern in a number of countries. Possibly because it has the most costly health service and because people there are not used to having to pay for other people's health care through taxes, the USA has been at the forefront of these worries. In particular, there has been concern about the unequal distribution of health finances between children and old people. For instance, it has been pointed out [62] that the prevalence of poverty in elderly people in the USA is less than the national average; for children it is substantially more. Federal expenditure on elderly people is six times that spent on children.

There have been suggestions as a result of the take up of health services, especially those in hospital, by elderly people that they are getting more than their fair share of health care. These arguments have been strongly resisted [63], but there have been suggestions that health and social care in the USA should be restricted for older people because during the 1960s and 1970s advocacy for and by elderly people in the USA resulted in a large number of federal programmes and created 'a welfare state for the elderly'.

This was brought about by extremely successful lobbying from a number of groups, most powerfully the American Association of Retired Persons, with 23 million members. The enormous membership was attracted by competitive rates for health and other insurance. Less powerful but more aggressive groups, such as the Gray Panthers may, by their use of the media, have had an effect in blowing away the myth of old age as one of peace and tranquillity. It is possible that the myth replacing it, one of selfish, grasping elderly people wresting resources from poor people and children, was a necessary concomitant. Some groups just cannot win 'imagewise'.

The government in Denmark has tried to limit the financial costs of caring for elderly people by developing community services. These took the form of home nurses and the provision of special housing for elderly people [64]. It has been suggested that it is cheaper to provide 30 hours a week of home care than to place an elderly person in an institution. The question remains whether the care is equivalent. In Germany, recent attempts have been made to reduce the admission of elderly people to hospital by providing home nursing, although it has proved difficult to bring about this change as people are more likely to feel that they are entitled to a specific type of care [65] because the system is insurance based. Similar problems have been met in Belgium, France, The Netherlands and Greece. Change has been a little easier to implement in countries that pay for their health care out of taxes as in Denmark, the UK, Italy and Sweden.

Austria has brought in compulsory financial support for relatives of frail elderly people living at home in order to limit the numbers admitted to hospital [66]. Most other European countries have tried to limit the use that people, especially older people, make of hospital beds. Similar pressures have caused New Zealand to adopt an internal market approach like the one in the UK, but the changes were brought in much more rapidly [67]. Here too emphasis has been on the development of primary care in an attempt to reduce the reliance of older people on hospital.

An important point, made originally about sub-Saharan Africa by one author, but equally true for all countries subject to marked variations in their economic well-being, is that in periods of economic decline countries reduce their payment for health services [68]. The interrelationship between wealth and health, especially for people on the edge of the economy, especially children, is such that this is the very time when more needs to be spent on health services to support such groups.

A favourite argument of those wishing to restrict care for elderly people is that they should not be allowed full access to high technology medicine, partly because it is assumed that high technology means admission to hospital and partly because of a general feeling that younger people are more deserving.

However, some authors have made the point [69] that increasing health care expenditure for elderly people is not particularly related to high technology intervention. Indeed medicine is, in reality, a low tech industry. It simply fusses about its high tech bits on television. The main costs in medicine are the expense of personnel, especially nurses, giving direct care. Restricting the use of high technology to younger people would therefore save very little. There is also an important argument which I have already mentioned, that people in the third age, no matter what their chronological age, appear to benefit as much as some young patients from complex treatment such as kidney dialysis, liver transplantation and heart transplantation.

Advocates of rationing resources in this way suggest that coercion will be necessary and that older people cannot be trusted to make wise choices about their own treatment. However, research work has shown that elderly people, when asked to make a choice about whether money should be allocated preferentially to the young or the old for instance, will make very similar choices to those of other generations [70] and are as keen as other age groups to protect children if there is to be any discrimination.

Pressures for change: economic

3

HEALTH CARE COSTS IN INDUSTRIAL COUNTRIES

Health care costs are a concern for every country. The country which spent most, the USA, spent almost 13% of its gross domestic product (GDP) on health care in 1990. This compares with 8–9% in Canada, France and Germany, and about 6% in Japan and the UK. In the USA, this percentage increased by nearly 3% each year in the 1980s [71].

There appears to be a relationship between the wealth of a country and the proportion of that wealth that it is willing to spend on health care. Figure 3.1 shows the figures for OECD countries in 1988. Richer countries (measured in GDP per person in dollar equivalents) spend a higher proportion of those riches on health. The countries above the line on the figure might be thought of as either getting less health services value for their money or being willing to spend more for health services than those below the line. It can be seen that some countries are well above the line, notably the USA. People in the UK often boast about the low cost of their health services, but as the figure shows, some of this difference is due to the relative poverty of the UK in the OECD family of countries.

However, there may be good news for the UK, because if spending on health is related to the wealth of a country, the UK is below the line in Figure 3.1. This suggests that either the UK gets its health services relatively cheaply when comparing like with like, or that it may be getting them too cheaply and the people of the UK are not treated well for the diseases they suffer. There is, of course, no way of knowing what the optimum level of spending is; the boundary between getting good health for the money invested and wasting it. We can get some clues by looking at the state of health in different countries, but the measures available are often not comparable between countries.

The people of the USA, at one extreme, each spent $2800 on health in 1990, nearly $1000 above the average for the other OECD countries. Health care

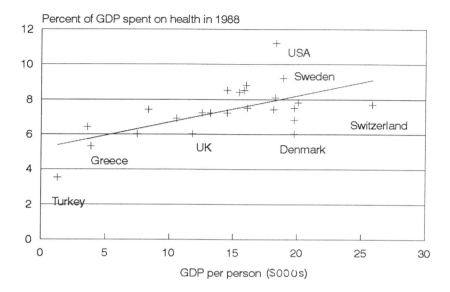

Figure 3.1 Wealthy countries spend more on health.

services also rose in price faster over the last two decades in the USA than in the other OECD countries. A number of private health insurers reimburse patients at different rates in the USA. This is expensive, especially in administrative costs. Administration costs about 15% of health expenditure in the USA, compared with 5% or less in the other OECD countries. If the USA reduced its administrative costs to the level in other developed countries, $80 billion a year could be saved, equivalent to about a third of total health spending for the developing countries.

Another reason for these very high health care costs may be that doctors in the USA are paid according to each service they provide and this is very expensive. Canada and Japan also pay their medical staff in this way, but they have developed methods of controlling how much their doctors spend. In Japan doctors check each others' costs, which holds down their colleagues' overspending. The tasks of doctors and other health workers are also set at a fixed cost. The Canadians also fix the price of the things that doctors and others do.

Countries which spend less, such as the UK, or which have not seen a rapid increase in the amount they spent in the last few years (Denmark, Germany and Sweden) tend to be those that put a ceiling on their pay to both doctors and hospitals. In the UK, the majority of primary care doctors (general practitioners) are paid a fee for each patient on their list. In Germany, although doctors are paid a fee for each task performed the fee is reduced if the number of services a doctor gives is above a set number. In Sweden, doctors are paid salaries.

There is another important point with regard to doctors' pay. They are usually the best paid professionals within a health system but, because they are relatively few in number, they cost, in terms of salaries, only a small proportion of the health budget. Nurses take up much more. However, it may not simply be the way that doctors earn their money, or the amount they get that makes a difference to overall costs. It may be the freedom that doctors have, or the extent to which they use that freedom, to dispose of the finances in the health service. They are the group that orders tests or therapy or bed rest for patients, all of which can cause marked variations in the costs of the health service.

In general, the developed OECD countries that have best contained the cost of health care are those with the most government control over health spending. Despite its relatively low level of spending, the UK government continues to make substantial changes to the administration of its health service with the aim of increasing its efficiency and restricting its spending.

The rise in costs of hospitals

The price of hospitals and other institutional care has been rising very rapidly in all developed countries. Figure 3.2 shows the price of health care for inpatient

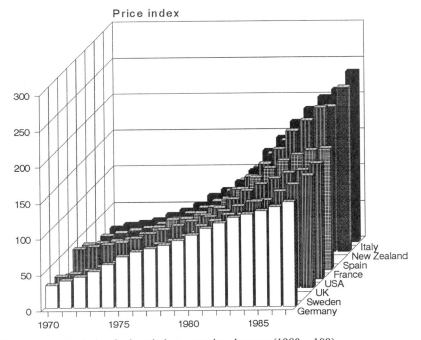

Figure 3.2 Price index for hospital care services by year (1980 = 100).

costs since 1970 in selected OECD countries. Prices in 1980 are shown as the index year with a value of 100, in order to counteract differences in currency inflation over the period.

All of the countries showed a marked rise in the price of their health costs. Interestingly, New Zealand, with one of the most extreme rises in costs, has felt driven to make rapid and extensive changes to the administrative structure of its health service by splitting it into two groups: purchasers of health services, who plan the service; and providers, who provide the care for patients.

The increase in the price of health care has not been confined to hospitals. Figure 3.3 shows the changes in prices for ambulatory medical care. There are three aspects to such care. First are the primary care services – the people who patients go to first when they have a problem, mainly general practitioners and a small number of others such as chiropodists. The second group of services are the outpatient services provided by specialists or secondary care givers, usually based in hospital. The third group are the community services, which traditionally give their care in the patient's home and consist mainly of district nurses, community psychiatric nurses, health visitors, chiropodists and, in some areas, therapists. More specialist groups are also developing in the community, such as nurses looking after diabetic patients or those with stomas.

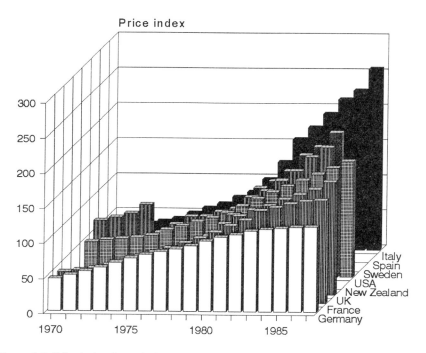

Figure 3.3 Price index for ambulatory care services by year (1980 = 100).

The figure for ambulatory services shows that they have increased, if anything, slightly more than the hospital services. Italy, in particular, has made a heavy investment in ambulatory services. For all of these areas, the UK has remained low on the list of price increases on health care.

There is a huge range in the overall amount spent on health care, with Switzerland spending nearly 50 times as much as Greece and Portugal. Countries which spend more than others on health services tend to spend it on both inpatient and ambulatory care. However, there are some differences. Spain spends less than a fifth of its total on ambulatory care, whereas Luxemburg spends almost two-thirds. In other words, Luxemburg puts much more emphasis on general practitioner, community based services and outpatient services than Spain. Figure 3.4 shows the data for the proportion spent on ambulatory care in OECD countries compared with the wealth of the different countries.

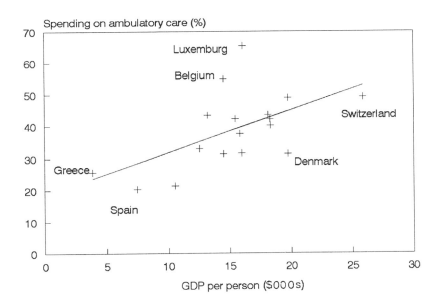

Figure 3.4 Richer countries spend a high proportion on ambulatory rather than hospital care.

Figure 3.4 shows that there is a trend for countries that are wealthier to spend a greater proportion of that wealth on ambulatory rather than hospital care. There are a number of possible reasons for this. It may be that the poorer countries within the OECD group are keen to ensure that secondary services, based around the hospital, are in place before the full development of primary and outpatient services. There may be strong pressure from the population for governments to develop acute general medical and surgical services first. The pressures for the treatment of emergencies as being of greatest priority has been well described by Illich [72] because labelling a problem as an emergency is one way, he describes, of ensuring that money will be spent on it, no matter how poor the country.

There will certainly be pressure from professional groups to invest money in hospital care. Most training, even today, is performed in hospital, even though the majority of doctors and a high proportion of other professionals in the medical field will spend their careers in community based or primary care. A further possibility is that pressures from urban, more politically aware popula-tions, who will also be more likely to benefit from hospital services, may be strongest in poorer countries, where the rural population has little voice. It is interesting that this tendency completely cuts across the World Health Organization policy of developing primary services first [73].

HEALTH SERVICES: GOOD VALUE FOR THEIR OUTCOMES?

We have seen that some countries spend much more than others on their health services. The central question, of what is the right amount is impossible to answer unless one has a clear view of what a health service is for. Health services are for a range of things, but some will be more important than others when judging their value for money. Health services:

- provide the service itself (e.g. consultations, operations)
- employ staff, thus having an effect on individuals and society
- have an effect on the country (e.g. fitter people)
- have an effect on patients (e.g. they live longer, feel better)

It is for us to choose which of these are the most important. Most people would say that the effect on patients or the population at large is the most important aspect of health services, including the hospital service. In general, the main effect one hopes for is that the population should live longer and have a better quality of life. Quality of life is not routinely measured in the UK, so we have to measure the success of health services overall by prolongation of life. This is very unsatisfactory, but for developed countries two main periods of life, when we are most at risk of death, are traditionally chosen: during the first year of life and the last years.

The first of these measures is the infant mortality ratio, the second is life expectancy. Life expectancy can be measured at a number of different times during one's life. In order to get an idea of the effect of services over the recent past, rather than a cumulative effect over a lifetime, I have chosen to look at life expectancy at the age of 60, rather than life expectancy at birth as a measure of what the health service is trying to achieve.

The question that we need to ask about these two outcome measures, these measures of success, is whether spending more on hospital services, rather than on the ambulatory (community care and general practitioner) services, gives better figures for the infant mortality ratio or life expectancy at 60 years. The data come from OECD countries. Figure 3.5 shows the numbers for infant mortality compared with the percentage spent on hospitals as contrasted with ambulatory services. The points on the scattergram show no real pattern, suggesting that the pattern of health service spending is not relevant to better infant mortality.

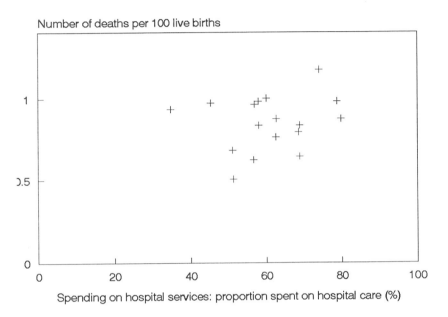

Figure 3.5 The proportion of care that is hospital based has no effect on infant mortality in OECD countries (each represented by a +).

Figure 3.6 shows similar numbers for life expectancy at 60 years of age in the OECD countries, for males and females separately. Once again there is no discernible pattern.

It appears that the amount a country spends on hospital, as distinct from its ambulatory, services has no effect on the main death rates. This suggests that, as far as death rates are concerned, a hospital orientated service is not better or worse than a community orientated one. Mortality rates do not reflect the work that health services do, whether hospital based or not. They are more closely related to the overall wealth of a nation than health spending [74].

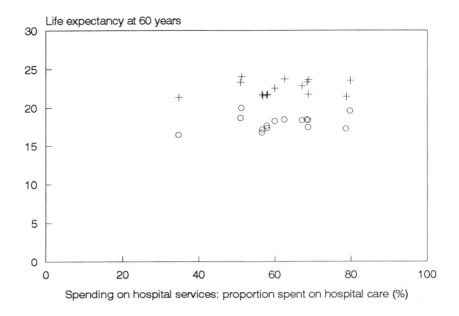

Figure 3.6 A higher proportion of spending on hospital care does not improve life expectancy at 60 years of age in OECD countries. Females (crosses); males (circles).

Costs of hospital staffing in the UK

In the UK, the hospital sector continues to absorb about two-thirds of the money put into health care annually. This has been changing over the years. Figure 3.7 shows the percentage increase in spending on the hospital and general practitioner sectors of the health service decade by decade since the NHS began [75].

It can be seen that the heyday of expansion for the hospital sector was in the 1960s as the district general hospitals were developing. Despite there now being fewer hospitals and beds, nearly a million people work in NHS hospitals in the UK. This has increased by more than three times since the founding of the health service. The number of beds for each staff member and the number of patients discharged per member of staff in hospitals fell steadily from the 1950s until the 1980s when the number rose a little. In other words, the service became more labour intensive until the 1980s. This, of course, will have increased the costs of hospitals.

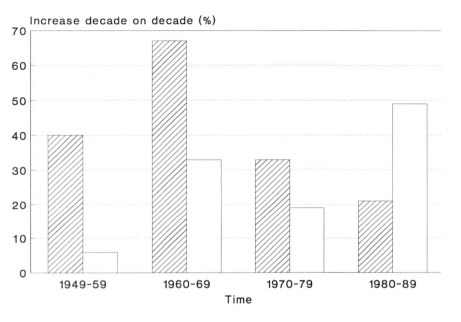

Figure 3.7 The heyday of hospital spending was in the 1960s. Spending adjusted to inflation. Hospital spending (shaded); general practice spending (unshaded). (Reproduced with permission from *Compendium of Health Statistics* (1989), 7th edn, Office of Health Economics, London.)

PUBLIC VIEWS ON THE AMOUNT TO BE SPENT

The demands on health services, especially if they are provided free at the point of access, as in the UK, are always greater than the supply [76]. There is a belief that society will not make difficult choices between demands for the money available, though this may be the perception of politicians wishing to run for election who do not even dare pose the question for fear of the answer they will get.

A sample survey of over 4000 people aged 17 and over in Cardiff, some years ago, did pose some relevant questions [77]. People were told how much was spent on the main services provided by the government in terms of how each pound, collected in taxes, was divided between those services. They were then asked if they would change the way the pound was divided.

Figure 3.8 shows the results for people of different ages, compared with the amount allocated to different services at present. It can be seen that the public in Cardiff wanted more spent on health, education, housing, the environment and transport and wanted the money to be taken from social security, to some extent, and to a greater degree from defence. People felt that the greatest redistribution should be from defence services into health services. The actual cost of the health service was 16p in the pound, whereas overall the people questioned felt that 20p in the pound should be allocated to health services.

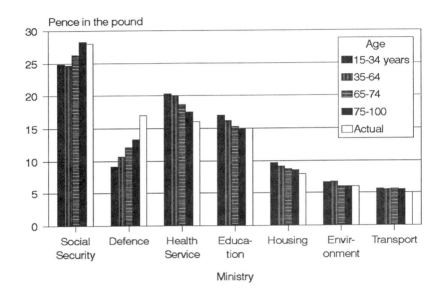

Figure 3.8 How different age groups would prefer to allocate their taxes.

The age groups were generally in agreement about which services should receive more money and which should get less. Older people were less radical in the degree of change they suggested. People aged 75 and over were in favour of more being spent on the health service but, curiously given their greater reliance on it compared with younger people, did not want to give as much as younger people. They may, remembering two world wars, have more feeling for the importance of defence services.

Slightly different results were seen if degree of disability rather than age was used to define the groups (Figure 3.9). The severely disabled were in favour of more spending on health services, housing, the environment and transport, at the cost of defence and social security. This is interesting, for some of the benefits paid in social security payments are intended for disabled people, though the system has often been criticized [57].

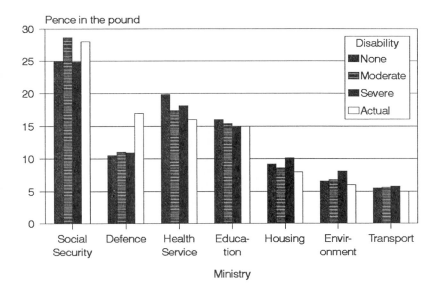

Figure 3.9 How people with disabilities would prefer to allocate their taxes.

Unfortunately this study did not ask where, within the health service, the money should be spent, though the group did have quite strong preferences about whom the money should be spent on if difficult choices had to be made.

ECONOMIC PRESSURES AND STRATEGIC PLANNING

The NHS and Community Care Act 1990 was brought in largely to restrict the expansion of spending on health care mentioned so far. The Act brought about the division of the health service into two groups: the purchasers and providers. The purchasers have developed from the district health authorities and are expected to have plans which are customized to their populations. At present these populations are mainly based on districts of about 200 000 people, but the districts are grouping together as commissions of about a million people. The task of the commissioners is to work out the special features of their particular areas and purchase health services to fit. The family health services authorities, so recently separated from the health authorities, are now being amalgamated into the new purchasing commissions. Regions in England have now been disbanded, being taken over by arms of central government, which will oversee the new system, particularly the development of provider trusts. The hospitals and community units have formed provider trusts, with their own boards of directors. These will provide the services to patients according to overall plans drawn up by the commissioners which are developed into contracts between the purchasers and the providers. There is therefore a degree of competition with other trusts to best fulfil the contract.

A robust approach to the purchaser's task of planning health services for a given population has been that of the Welsh Health Planning Forum, which, in Wales, acts as the health service arm of the central government department, the Welsh Office. As regional authorities have been disbanded in England the approach may form a template for the development of services elsewhere in the UK [78]. The English *Health of the Nation* document has proposed a similar approach.

These documents have produced a number of broad principles and some more detailed guidance which has filled out the details of the government's policy. Firstly, there is to be much more flexibility between primary prevention, primary care and secondary care, meaning that more money is to be spent on prevention and primary care. Secondly, patients should be treated as close to their own homes as is feasible, meaning more use of general practitioner services for such things as minor surgery. Thirdly, budgets for working in this way will be distributed to those working in the field, as far as possible. There is an assumption that such moves will ensure that services are more efficient and that there will be an incentive for the services to save money, which can then be diverted to improving or further developing that service.

The Forum, in a document designed to develop more ideas in the same direction, suggests that the great majority of people needing acute general surgery could be cared for on a day basis. Acute general medicine and geriatrics, apart from the intensive care services, could, without any new knowledge, be carried out at home or in small localized community units. Such a move, it is suggested, would meet with the approval of patients and be no less costly to the health service than the present system. This is because the money spent would be used to pay for direct care; there would be no need to provide all of the extremely expensive hotel and maintenance services provided by hospitals because the patient would be in his or her own home or in a small homely unit. The care provided by other services, especially social services, would be paid for separately [79], whereas in hospital all services provided on the premises, whether part of health care or not, are provided free.

One of the problems with attempting to bring about such changes in the past has been that health services are so big that they are difficult to change. The NHS is the tenth largest employer in Europe and trying to alter the way it provides services has been likened to manipulating a supertanker. Any changes that need to be made take such a long time to put in place that one may have changed one's mind by the time they happen.

Part of the development of purchasers and providers in the UK health service is a commitment to change, to follow whatever the contract set up by the purchasers says. The NHS and Community Care Act thus brings into being a 'managed internal market' in health services. One effect will be to speed up the changes away from hospital care towards community and home based care as suggested by government policy.

The effect of the internal market on hospitals

There are many types of 'managed internal market' throughout the world, each with different approaches, different external limits and different methods of funding. In the UK, each purchasing group, originally the district health authority, is based on a geographical area and is given funds according to the population in that area. The amount given may be varied according to a formula, for instance if the population is deprived or has high levels of sickness there may be some extra money.

Each health authority decides which providers to purchase its services from. These may be hospital or community based trusts within the health service, or they may buy services for their population from private or voluntary suppliers. In practice the first providers to be approached have been those in the same area, which, before the split into purchasers and providers, were managed directly by the health authority. This is especially so for community based services where the local service providers are already part of the community that requires help.

The authority can, however, ask general practitioners to refer patients to services anywhere in the country if the cost and quality of the service is much better than that provided locally. At the moment the threat of going to another provider has been used more as a lever to improve the cost or quality of a local service, or to bring about changes in a service, for example towards a more community orientated mental illness service, than directly to close down a provider. Where hospital and community trusts appear not to be able to manage within their budgets, either because of poor accounting or because they have a bad reputation, successful trusts have tended to take over their functions.

Hospital based trusts provide mainly acute medical and surgical inpatient services. They can therefore be put under much greater pressure by purchasers than community and longer term services because their patients are more mobile and can therefore be referred elsewhere. In addition, the service providers are entrenched in a large stock of buildings. Hospital trusts therefore have a wider range of competitors in other hospitals and will attempt to reduce their costs for each patient. This will result in shorter lengths of stay and more day care. In addition, the community based trusts will be keen to try to take some of the lucrative acute care medical work using hospital at home or day care schemes, or, by collaborating with general practitioners, to move some of the work traditionally done by secondary services into primary care.

In the UK, the purchasers are able to obtain only state funds for purchasing.

The health authority and trust board members are directly chosen by the Secretary of State and are therefore, in effect, both an arm of government. This is in contrast to the health maintenance organizations (HMOs) in the USA, where private insurance and personal payments can be made to the organizations.

Health authorities are being grouped together as purchasing consortia, which bring together a number of health authorities with family health service authorities, who have the overall responsibility of managing general practitioner and dental services. The new consortia oversee populations of around one million people. One effect of these larger groups for purchasing is that there will be a greater number of hospital and community trusts within a given geographical area. There will therefore be less of a tendency for purchasers to favour 'their own' hospitals and automatically purchase from the nearest trust. This will allow consortia to force more rapid changes in the service, if they so wish.

General practitioner fundholders

General practitioners in group practices with over 5000 patients may apply to become fundholding general practitioners. They are given a budget, based on their previous custom, which is estimated to cover the costs of admitting their patients to hospital for routine work, in practice mainly for routine surgery, their use of community based services, and their drug and staff costs. The system is intended to reduce unnecessary referrals by general practitioners to hospital and to encourage general practitioners to extend the amount and nature of the work that they can absorb themselves. General practitioners in practices with over 3000 patients may receive community services, drugs and staff costs only.

The aim is to reduce the amount of hospital care that general practitioners use. In order to help them do this they are allowed to absorb a proportion of any savings they make into the practice. In fact, general practitioners in the UK do not seem to be particularly bad at referring patients inappropriately to secondary care [80] but presumably there is always a margin which can be increased towards general practitioner care. They are also allowed to employ staff to develop the number of procedures that they can carry out within the surgery or in the patient's home. A third aspect which general practitioners are expected to manage themselves is their drug costs. They are given a budget for this and are expected to keep within it.

General practitioners are therefore purchasers of some services; about four-tenths of the total budget for a given group of patients. Emergency services are purchased in the great majority of places by health authorities. Some practices are still resistant to becoming fundholders and special arrangements will have to be made for small practices, though some pilot projects for collecting together such general practitioners are underway.

Some attempts are being made to allow experienced general practitioners to purchase all services for their patients, including emergency care. If this idea spreads throughout the country it will make the health authority purchasers, in effect, redundant as far as setting contracts for services for the population is concerned. They will have only a strategic planning and monitoring task to ensure that the multiplicity of general practice purchasers were following some kind of general plan.

There are moves within health authorities, which possibly see the writing on the wall for their future, to make plans for the health care for populations, within the authority, in small areas, of about 50 000 people, based on the local general practices, and, wherever possible, using common boundaries between the health authorities and social services departments. The point of these moves has been to try to customize the primary care, community and non-health services, such as social work, housing and education for the particular locality. In this way they hope to be able to offer general practitioners services that more closely follow the local needs of the population. This may be a way of giving the benefits of fundholding to general practitioners who are not fundholders – allowing them a say in the health authority contract with hospitals and community trusts in order to obtain the quality of care they want, without the problem of having to balance their books.

Provider competition

The essence of the managed market in the UK is that there is competition between the NHS trusts the public providers, private health providers and others, including voluntary and self-help groups for the health authority's finance [81]. The NHS trusts [82] have been set up, especially in their system of capital funding, so that they do not have a natural advantage over other providers who are not within the health service. However, the NHS trusts are several orders of magnitude bigger than the private and voluntary providers. On the social side of community care the government has gone so far as to insist that a high proportion of the money to be spent on community care must be spent with the independent sector. This has been a big problem for some social services departments wishing to provide home care. Some social services departments have spent a great deal of effort persuading, funding and even inventing voluntary groups so that services will be available for them to purchase. It is to be hoped that such efforts will result in a wider range of services than has been provided in the past.

Patient choice

Patients are expected to exercise a choice of what services they want through their general practitioner who is expected to act as their advocate in finding the best quality services with, for instance, the lowest waiting lists. It is assumed that the issues of quality are not well enough understood by potential patients for them to make wise choices on their own. The patients can, if they wish, freely change their general practitioner if he or she is not proving to be a good advocate.

The reforms produce a balance between choice, spending and quality in different ways. Purchasers limit patient choice by regulating how much they will pay. They increase it by some competition between providers for contracts because a wise purchaser will not buy all of one service with one provider, to maintain that element of choice. As a result, providers with similar costs will be expected to increase the quality of their service to attract patients [83].

Purchasers are committed to buying in services more selectively than in the past. They can now put pressure on providers to follow more closely their own strategic aims and government policy. It is also hoped that the system will allow the service to get away from the priorities set by those who, in the past, were simply keen to develop highly technical secondary care of dubious benefit for patients, but with high publicity value. This included types of organ transplant, complex cardiac surgery in the newborn and highly technical approaches to infertility.

Purchasers, if they are to be successful, will concentrate on solving problems that are solvable, often using reasonably simple primary care services, which are often those that will provide improving health for their population. It is known, for instance that minor trauma to fingers causes a huge proportion of days lost off work. Concentrating on the prevention of such injuries and improving the skills of the surgery given by nurses or junior doctors might well prove extremely rewarding in terms of better health for citizens and the economy of the country. Such a policy is unlikely, however, to appear on any television programme; nor will anyone be made a professor as a result.

The pressure for costly new treatment

It is not just luck that simple problems, simply solved are the most cost effective; nor that such solutions are not given a high priority. The pressures on health services to develop new approaches have come, in the main, from a combination of the medical profession and industry developing complex equipment or drugs. The pressure to find new solutions is fed, on the one hand, by professionals and their need to do research into new methods, and on the other by private industry requiring to develop new markets.

The medical profession is under a number of pressures to discover new methods of applying knowledge. Part of the pressure is the development of the doctor as scientist. The role model for medical students is the professor of medicine or surgery, chosen mainly on the record of his or her scientific, as distinct from medical, work. A young doctor in training will be in fierce competition with others for the next step up the ladder. As virtually all of the serious competitors will have the necessary postgraduate qualifications, the way in which a graduate will be able to stand out will be by owning one or more research degrees and by the number of published scientific papers he or she has published.

Population health status and needs

Improving health revolves around improving the length of someone's life and the quality of life he or she can achieve, if a particular treatment is given. It may, of course, slow down the rate of deterioration. If the treatment or care does none of these things there is no point in it. There is a competitive aspect to improving health. Some treatments or care will provide more health than others and if there is not enough money for both, the one providing most must be chosen.

Purchasing the services that give most improvement in health is therefore quite likely to cut across the development of new scientific discoveries. New approaches, unless they are stunningly effective from the first, are not likely to provide more improvements in health than old, tried and tested methods for a number of years. Indeed no discoveries, apart from the discovery of antibiotics in the 1930s and 1940s, have been so obviously effective that they did not need careful evaluation. There needs to be a mechanism for the evaluation of such new ideas so that important advances are not ignored.

The difficulty is that virtually all new treatments are hailed as a break-through, particularly when being marketed by a private company, often in conjunction with a group of doctors who are gathering research material on the subject as qualifications for their next job. One of the difficulties of purchasing only treatment or care that provides improved health is that it is necessary to have information about both the prevalence and severity of illness, and of the other circumstances associated with bad health, such as poor housing, poverty and unemployment.

There is a problem here, for often the social conditions of patients exacerbate the effect of the disease process to such an extent that the most effective intervention may be to alter their social conditions. This may make the health service and its interventions irrelevant or, at least, relatively unimportant, compared with the other pressures. The benefit of the purchaser provider system in the NHS is that purchasing money can be more easily diverted more freely to non-health service interventions than in the past.

Deciding on what is effective

There is no point in purchasing treatments or services that do not work. It is often difficult to get good proof that many of the generally accepted treatments used in the health service, especially the older ones, do work. Some health education or preventive services are very effective. If a person already has a disease or illness his or her health will improve if he or she is cured or the progress of the disease is slowed down. However, the cure may be temporary, may have side-effects that reduce health, or may simply prevent or reduce further deterioration.

The cost of treatments or care services varies enormously. Purchasers need to know the cost effectiveness of different interventions in the individual case and,

for populations, for each condition or health problem. In addition, it is not justi-
fiable to buy in very expensive services that are not very effective when other
treatments that are more cost effective can be bought.

Social values

A third, often ignored part of purchasing for health is the value that the general
public puts on different groups. There are different ways to do this, but there are
democratic and ethical reasons to involve the public in these decisions. Some
evaluations include measures of social value when judging the benefits of treatments. However, there are many health decisions that can only be decided by
choices which need public debate. It is likely that if the public is given more
choice in the services it can use, people will tend to prefer those which are more
locally provided, as long as they are equally effective. The system will therefore
be biased away from large centralized hospitals towards local care.

PURCHASING IMPROVED HEALTH – PROBLEMS SO FAR

A large number of papers have been written on the first few years of the UK
reforms and these have been well summarized [84]. When the new approach
was set up there was no tradition for people in the UK health service to measure
the costs of individual services or to try to measure their quality objectively.
There had been an assumption that the job of the health service was to bring
together patients and professionals who were suitably trained and let them get
on with it. Costs were usually collected across specialties and by function. That
is, the cost of employing nurses was calculated separately from the costs of
doctors, the costs of pathological tests separately from the cost of the laundry
service. For this reason it was difficult to see where the main expenses of any
one service lay.

It was therefore very difficult to decide what a case of appendicitis, for
instance, cost to treat. Neither was there a means of deciding if patients were
getting better treatment from one professional or another, short of a large
number of complaints made by patients about a particular service or some kind
of gross misconduct. Information that has been collected emphasizes the enormous variation in the cost of different services, whether an operation or treatment for a disease, from place to place. Even less information is available about
the needs of different groups in an area, though it was known in general terms
that the poor and unemployed were likely to use more services than average
[85] and that black people tended not to use the available services fully [86].

Early attempts by purchasers to obtain information about what people in their
area needed had to rely on the providers that they were evaluating to provide it,
as well as information about whom general practitioners referred to for treatment. General practitioner referrals are still one way that purchasers can predict

the demands that patients are likely to make on the secondary services, in the community or in hospital. This has the disadvantage of maintaining the existing system of referral, without knowing whether the referral was because of or despite giving a good service. In addition, people with problems may not be referred by general practitioners, or may be unwilling to visit the general practitioner in the first place because of his or her poor service.

UK purchasing authorities are gradually learning how to use the system for the advantage of their patients. Early on, purchasing authorities set up 'block contracts'. This in effect meant paying for a similar service to previous years, with some adjustment for the way the service had been progressing, with an amount added on for inflation. Block contracts have been used mostly for large essential services where the workload varies greatly, such as casualty departments.

In cost and volume contracts, where there are higher transaction costs (i.e. costs in setting up the contract itself) providers can increase their throughput to free some capacity for other contracts. Transaction costs are even higher in the third method used for buying in services, the cost per case contract. This is rarely, despite the name, the cost of caring for a single patient worked out according to what services he or she used. Such an approach is extremely expensive, and unnecessary where individuals are not billed directly. More commonly, information on what was wrong with a patient is collected and standard tables of relative costs, drawn up originally in the USA, are available for deciding what to pay for the group of patients with that condition. This information is based on groupings related to the original diagnosis of the patient, known as diagnosis related groups.

The tables give relative, not actual costs so that they need to be re-calculated in money terms in different countries or different areas where the overall costs of services may be more or less expensive. In this way, given the case mix, that is the sorts of diseases and problems patients come in with, the likely costs incurred by one unit, compared with another can be calculated. The system is quite complex to administer and not completely accurate so that some trusts, reimbursed in this way will be relatively well off, others relatively poor.

Experience in other countries, especially the USA, has suggested that some hospitals will learn to use the system to their own advantage, such as by reclassifying patients with simple appendicitis into complicated appendicitis when only minor complication may be present, thus moving patients into the higher cost band. This can often be difficult to detect for much of the information on which the system depends has to come from the provider.

So far, since the development of the UK internal market, there is little evidence of increased efficiency or saving of money. There has been some increase in administrative costs. The number of accountants in the NHS between 1987 and 1991 rose from 2500 to 4000, and costs attributed to general management salaries went up tenfold over the same 4-year period from £25 million to £251 million. Some of these increases reflect a change in the way that senior nurses were paid, as they moved onto the management structure. It is typical of the problems which beset the system that these differences cannot be separated out. On the other hand, there is evidence for the first time of the enormous cost differences between hospitals for the same operation, which should, in time, bring costs down overall [87].

A general problem is that, in the short term, the cost of contracting may be greater than the reductions brought about by greater efficiency and choice. It is possible that this will be true in the long term as well. The costs of regulation and the economic and management costs of developing contracts may be higher than the benefits of savings from efficiency and productivity gains. Pressure to change the way that services are provided will therefore be considerable.

The evidence is that there are considerable differences between health authority and general practitioner purchasing [88]. There is little evidence so far of the new system being exploited by providers, though the weakening of the purchaser function, by marked reductions in the numbers of purchasers, the development of consortia as purchasers, covering populations of about a million people and the removal of the regional tier may allow such exploitation in future.

There are a number of possible ways providers can do this. Patients could be treated as emergencies, not planned admissions, to get higher payments on a cost per case basis. Furthermore, patients may be kept in hospital longer to charge for extra days where the hospital has excess capacity. Repeated admissions may be used for a single patient who has multiple needs with the patient discharged each time so that the hospital can charge each time the patient is readmitted. Providers may discharge patients early into the community or to other services to save costs.

Purchasing authorities have been so busy learning the new process of deciding the health needs of the people in their populations, setting priorities and developing contracts [89] that the niceties of contracting for improved health have not really been approached. If the system is to work it will need to develop on a long-term basis. The real cost advantages may well not begin to be visible until considerable changes in the way that health services are delivered are brought about.

The internal market may be a better way of making sure that there are overall improvements in the health of the population, which is the responsibility of the purchaser, because of the freedom that they have to move services away from hospitals. Services given in general practice and other parts of the primary care team can be provided more flexibly than in large hospitals. This approach is much less easy for providers to manipulate, especially as patients will be more aware of what they are receiving on an individual basis. Fundholding general practitioners, without the large numbers of patients to deal with that have restricted the action of health authorities, have been more demanding in purchasing their care from both hospital and community providers than the purchasers have been to date.

The more serious problem in the future may be that health authority purchasers will have views about which services provide most health improvements. The method of measuring this is not so precise that, even with the best will in the world, general practitioners are all likely to ask for the same services at the same level of quality. Without goodwill some general practitioners might decide to avenge old scores by asking for quality or other standards which will severely try the ability of a provider to deliver the service. In addition, health authorities, over the years, have been quite closely guided by different government policies on the way that some services should develop. An example is in the move to community care for mentally ill people. It is not clear, at present, how such policy decisions will constrain individual general practitioner fundholders [88].

There is a tendency to assume that only health authorities will purchase services aimed specifically at improving health, and that general practitioners are incapable or uninterested in doing so. However, if a choice has to be made, primary and community based health care are more promising than hospital care for improving health. The merger of health authorities with family health service authorities means that the joint commissioners have closer links with general practitioners. This may be enough for them to be able to put pressure on fundholding general practitioners to keep in line with the strategy set out by the authorities.

Trusts are increasing their competitiveness and one of the main factors in this will be their ability to deliver better health status for their patients. However, trusts are very dependent on meeting their financial targets which may or may not force them into practices which promote overall patient well-being. The task of the purchasers is to try to see that they are guided this way [84].

In the USA, payment for services is usually made on a cost for each case basis. The actual services used are identified and costed. There are very large costs involved in this process [90]. Safeguards are needed to avoid expensive and unnecessary procedures being used. In the USA, one pressure towards choosing the most expensive option is the fear of litigation. There is a feeling that an expensive, rather than a simpler cheap approach, is more likely to satisfy patients or their relatives.

Means of improving health must include the social values and the priorities the local population put on different problems. The challenge is to involve the public in debating and setting priorities. One way is to have elected representatives running the health authority, as in Sweden. However, the Swedish Counties do not have a good record of deciding on priorities. As often happens, lay elected people tend to give a great deal of influence to the academic professionals who are developing new treatments. The problem here is that exciting new high tech ideas are also popular, leading to extensive media coverage. Lay representatives may find it difficult to make rationing decisions when those who will lose out by the decision will have a voice in the next election. There is also the difficult decision to be made when the public decides that something that does not lead to improved health should still be purchased.

IS NON-HEALTH INVESTMENT MORE EFFECTIVE?

I have shown that medical interventions in general do not seem to have a great deal of effect on the widest measures of the health of nations, at least not in the developed nations. There is evidence that the main factors influencing, for instance, the infant mortality rate in a country have more to do with the wealth of that country in general terms than the amount spent on the health services. Recent work has suggested that high unemployment and greater inequalities in wealth have extensive effects on the health of individuals in small areas of the UK [91].

The obvious approach to improving health in such communities is to try to improve rates of employment and reduce financial inequalities. Within the health service, however, it is likely that at least some of these untoward effects can be helped, as long as the service is capable of customizing the assistance it provides to take these large differences in small areas into account. Primary and community based care is more likely to be effective in these circumstances, wherever it is feasible to provide it.

4

Pressures for change: technological

THE DEVELOPMENT OF TECHNOLOGICAL CHANGES

The full development of new scientific knowledge in medicine, depends on:

- the existence of knowledge which can be applied
- people with the skills to apply the knowledge
- social and political acceptability of the advance
- financial backing for its development
- marketing skills for the development
- financial backing for widespread manufacture.

The main point to be made is that the existence of such knowledge, in itself, is only a step in the numerous processes which need to be sifted and to be favourable for the knowledge to be used. The speed of development of scientific ideas and making them into useful and saleable products is affected by social, economic and political conditions. The development of most modern technologies requires money and, in the majority of cases, a lot of it. The social and political stimuli for the development of new ideas appear to be increasing in their effect. An important spur appears to be the increase in communications, especially television, which, in turn, promotes change. The media tend to support an exaggerated view of science and scientific discovery which suggests that each new study is a breakthrough and every new product will be a success. This appears to have led to a belief that virtually all medical problems are understood and a notion that there is a technical answer to all of those problems.

Pressures to apply new technology

The relationship between the public and new technology is variable. In some instances, far from being worried by new developments the public seems to have a fascination with new ideas. Research looking at whether patients are worried about being admitted to high technology, intensive care units has shown variable results. Some researchers suggest that patients are disturbed by these methods of treatment, others suggest that patients having such care believe that they are 'getting the best' [92].

At the same time there has been an increasing demand from part of the general public for a movement towards holistic and alternative medicines. These embody different attitudes towards technology, and emphasize the whole person, rather than the physiological, aspects of therapies. This suggests that some groups of people are growing sceptical about the claims of the medical industry.

There is a spin off to this interest in a social approach to medicine, which has been taken up by the mainstream medical services. This is found in the health promotion groups which wish to encourage people to take more control over the prevention and treatment of their own illnesses. This usually involves a process of education so that people more fully understand illness, its therapy and the methods of prevention. The medical professionals, doctors and nurses, have not traditionally been taught how to teach or even to make their meaning clear to others. There has not even, until recently, been any attempt to choose medical professionals who have a natural aptitude for working with other people, either colleagues or patients.

The approach I was taught was that the best way of obtaining a history of illness from a patient was to 'remain on the gentlemanly side of aggression'. This involved firing a series of questions at the patient to elicit a diagnosis, without having to engage in a rambling chat which, left to themselves, most patients were prone to do. The latter took much more time and considerably extended the number of possible diagnoses that one had to take into account. As the aim was to end up with one diagnosis this was assumed to be a bad idea.

Those days are going. However, good communication is not enough; people must also be aware of what can really be expected from technological advances. Citizens of the USA are better informed on medical matters than those of any other country, yet they also appear to be the most demanding in terms of a 'pill for every ill'. This appears to be part of a conspiracy where the public demands answers to impossible questions of doctors who promise not to tell them that there are no satisfactory answers as long as they continue to demand their services.

More realistic presentation of the possibilities which medical technology has to offer would be an important step forward. This requires close questioning of some of the media-prone medical establishments about whether people actually get better, or remain no worse for their new wonder therapy and whether simple and effective procedures could have been obtained for the same price. One sometimes has to wait considerable periods for the answers to such questions, which is a disadvantage when the tabloids want answers by their evening deadline.

PROBLEMS OF HIGH TECHNOLOGY

Generally, despite the fuss made about it, health services use very little high technology. Over two-thirds of the budget of most health services goes on staffing costs. Yet there is a danger in the rapid development of technology, for health care can become over reliant on trying to alter those aspects of illness which can best be altered by the technology. There is often, within the health professions, an inadequate understanding of the limits of machines and the information they generate. Nurses and doctors are often given new facilities and instructions to 'watch that machine' without understanding, for instance, that abnormal pattern recognition can only be maintained for a maximum of 20 minutes, so that a shift system for watching cardiac monitors is essential [93]. An increasing reliance on machines may also lead to a loss of some human skills. However, experience with some machines, for example in echocardiography, has consistently underlined the accuracy of the newer diagnostic tool when compared with the stethoscope, the original diagnostic tool.

There have been complaints that high technology medicine has led doctors to be less caring and more concerned with the diseased organ or tissue than the person as a whole. However, these are not new complaints and are more related to the way that doctors are selected, trained and given their role models than the increasing use of high technology. High technology approaches have little to offer many disease entities and rarely affect the social and psychological aspects which are always important and often critical to the recovery of patients. Social and psychological support may also help to protect people against some diseases or restrict their effects

Pressure on the health services to use new technology has often been driven by industry where developing these technologies may be a spin off from other work. Critics of the over-reliance some health professionals place on high technology have suggested [94] that better control of a small number of risk factors, which are directly under the control of patients themselves, could prevent almost half of all deaths in people under retirement age and a large proportion of cases of chronic disease. The changes required would be largely to do with altering people's behaviour and would not require any high technology intervention.

An important criticism of technology is that it diverts planning and other resources and, perhaps most importantly, attention, away from simple but effective interventions, while at the same time being relatively inefficient itself. If there is to be reasonable equality in terms of the amount of health care given to people then high cost, high technology care to a small number must also be called into question [95]. In the USA, for instance, the top 1% of users of medical care use up just under one-third of all health care spending, the top 5% use up half. Patients with chronic renal disease are a quarter of one percent of the population in the USA but spend a tenth of the Medicare budget (for poor people) in the USA. This is largely due to the cost of the high technology intervention that disease requires and to the high staffing levels needed to maintain such machinery.

In developed countries there is still a strong belief and commitment to the idea that medicine will progress and give us increasing power over disease. This suggests that we will ultimately be able to control the disease processes and that this control will come about through new inventions. It is a curious belief, fostered by medical professionals to some extent and popularized by the media who seem constantly to be looking for magic. The therapies developed, although often welcomed by many of the general public, are rarely demanded by them. I have mentioned that the main advocates for technological development in medicine are the medical profession and the pharmaceutical industry. Cardiac transplantation was not demanded by the public nor was it the result of a public campaign. Once developed, however, media attention, with its tendency to dramatize, increased demand among physicians, patients and industry to develop new and better methods.

The initial development of a new, complex treatment often puts patients at high risk while the method is perfected. It is true that patients chosen for such risky therapy are usually mortally ill, but that simply makes the whole process more macabre. Once developed, it is assumed that the new approach, no matter what the cost, will be available for all. The future for disabled people is assumed to be the bionic person – half machine, half human – rather than someone who is adjusted, both internally and by a friendly environment, to be able to manage a reasonably normal life despite his or her disabilities. The latter is less media worthy, but much more likely to work and, perhaps most importantly, commits everyone to the idea that disabled people can cope and that it is their right to live in a community that allows them to cope.

Once a new therapy is developed, politicians and voluntary health groups often join the bandwagon, eager to take some of the credit for the breakthrough. Voluntary organizations, directly aware of the horrors of a particular disease through clients and family members, will advocate that more money should be given to that particular group. They often fund further research in the hope that it will come up with some new technology to cure the particular disease central to the group's interest.

A high tech answer, which will remove the disease entity, has no connotations of blame, and is therefore preferred to simple preventive or palliative research. A good example of this occurred a couple of years ago when a charity working on behalf of arthritis sufferers closed down work on the measurement and treatment of pain in these patients to follow a highly speculative path on the cellular basis of, and possibly the cure of, rheumatoid arthritis. At least four such cures have been announced for rheumatoid arthritis in the past 20 years but none has lasted for more than 6 months.

Another example of the influence of voluntary organizations is seen when people collect money for complex equipment. A common recent example has been to buy magnetic resonance imaging (MRI) scanners. These are often presented with great pomp to the local hospital which then has to choose whether to reject the gift or to try to find the running costs to keep it going. One of the dangers of the new internal market within the health service will be that providers who have available to them large quantities of technological equipment will press for this to be used in order to pay for the costs it engenders.

New drugs and medicines are the centre of a huge and important industry. There is, as with all technological developments, a danger of providing new ideas or products with minimal or no improvement over the old ones. The competitiveness of the drug companies, in particular, puts pressure on them to provide the market with new drugs for which a premium can be charged. Unless they do this they will not be able to keep up the momentum of the research, development and marketing cycle they have got into.

Apart from drugs, there are a number of therapeutic advances which will be important to the development of medicine over the coming decade. Lasers are used in a number of ways, especially with small tubes (endoscopes and even narrower catheters) down which they may be passed to many parts of the body that were previously only accessible through major surgery. The laser can be used to cut and cauterize diseased tissues. This is useful in many parts of medicine and surgery, and in some cases is already reasonably tested against the existing treatment.

I have mentioned the financial pressures that the demand for health care causes in a country. One of the factors causing such pressures is the cost of researching and developing the technology itself. The cost of development makes it difficult for some new technologies to get on to the market, though costly products sometimes seem to get accepted simply because other health groups have one. It has been suggested that new technology accounts for a quarter of the increased expenditure on health that developed nations have seen over the past two decades [96]. The problem for the UK is subtly different from that in countries which rely on a private insurance system for paying health bills. In insurance based systems the new technology may be too expensive for it to be accepted by some insurers, or they may require higher premiums. This leads to two tiers of service, divided by the wealth of the patients. In the UK, new technological advances usually develop in teaching hospitals and are then gradually picked up by other districts. This leads to differences in availability depending on where patients live, their willingness to travel to the centre of excellence and, an important and unusual characteristic of British doctors, a rationing of the new service towards younger and middle class patients.

TECHNOLOGY AND HOSPITALS: SCANNING

Much of the development of high technology within medicine has been aimed at outlining structures inside the body without having to break the skin and therefore without pain. X-rays were the first of these, and were especially useful for outlining bony structures. This was followed by the use of ultrasound, used in situations where X-rays were likely to be harmful, especially in pregnant women. X-rays can be used in conjunction with radio-opaque substances to outline parts of the body but the equipment is costly. In recent years, new imagers and scanners have increased in cost. It remains to be seen if they have also increased in terms of their usefulness.

The first of these, the computed tomography (CT) scanner, appeared in 1972, and began the development of systems for holding information in computers, rather than on film or photographs. New imaging methods that use such data include the CT scanner, MRI and the positron emission tomography (PET) scanner. The benefit of keeping information in a digital format on a computer is that it can be accurately transmitted along phone or data lines and will, at the end of the process, be as accurate as it was originally [97]. The data can be transmitted anywhere there is a telephone line and the image reproduced on a computer at the other end. Therefore, although the process has to be undertaken in hospital, the results can be sent to any other location, such as to the general practitioner's surgery.

These machines are able to give images of cross-sections of the tissues of the body and are said to be most useful where there are abnormal growths, such as cancer, or abnormal spaces such as cysts, or where parts of a structure have been disrupted, such as in joints. Some can give a three-dimensional image, which is useful for complex structures.

The CT scanner gives quite a high dose of radiation to the patient being studied and for this reason, and because of the development of MRI scanning, it has been used less recently. They have in common that they are extremely expensive and are being very strongly marketed. They give interesting pictures, especially the MRI scanner, of places that are sometimes impossible to explore safely. It would seem self evident that such equipment would be tested in detail before huge financial outlays are made on it. However, the studies made on their effectiveness have been quite small in number and extremely uncritical. There is a desperate need for the systems to be evaluated against the best alternative methods.

Measuring the effectiveness of MRI

MRI needs to be carried out in hospital. The equipment is very large and needs the back-up services of a department of medical imaging costing about £1 million in capital terms and having revenue consequences of about £500 000 each year thereafter. The equipment is still developing and will therefore become obsolete in between 5 and 10 years. This is a huge cost outlay for any part of the health service and obviously needs to be examined carefully to make sure that the method gives sufficient improvements for patients to justify the costs.

MRI has a number of theoretical advantages. It is safe, in that it does not expose patients to ionizing radiation, as do CT scanners and X-rays. There is no need to inject any substance into the body to show the structures more clearly. (A number of techniques, such as angiography and myelography, require such an injection with some attendant dangers to patients who may be allergic to the substance injected.) The image can be taken in any direction and recently three-dimensional imaging has been possible. This allows one to look at the relation-ships between different parts of the body and, in effect, to look at the internal structure.

MRI is particularly useful for obtaining good images of the skull and brain, particularly in patients with multiple sclerosis and in children with gross congenital abnormalities of the brain. It can also give good images of the spinal column. MRI is also useful for looking at the details of joints. Given the things that it can do it may seem extraordinary that is has not been proved to be unequivocally cost effective, for at least one of its many functions. The reasons for this lie with the relationship between new developments and the diagnosis, treatment and effectiveness of medical practice.

However, there are a number of basic rules when comparing the cost and effectiveness of new technology [98]:

- the options to be compared must be clearly defined
- there must be straightforward measures of effectiveness
- the background to the analysis must not be expected to change.

The use of MRI is not covered by these criteria, which makes it very diffi-cult to evaluate the method. Some people have attempted to look critically at the use of MRI [99], but no studies have yet produced reliable evidence to show that the method is cost effective even for diagnostic use in a particular organ or part of the body. This has not stopped MRI scanners from spreading rapidly throughout the developed world. As with most studies into the effec-tiveness of new technology in medicine, the early work was very poor in that it was uncritical, comparisons between different methods were often badly made and the outcome for patients was not properly described. A good image, especially in colour, was considered an end in itself rather than assessing whether such imaging led to a better result for the patient. In a review of eight studies of MRI [100] all but six were found to contain basic methodological errors.

Another review [101] applied the accepted criteria for research methods:

- evidence of research planning
- appropriately used sensitivity and specificity
- appropriate presentation of the data
- good calculation of the values
- comparison with a gold standard
- a randomized controlled trial
- interpretation of results carried out 'blind'

- measurement of inter-observer variability
- correct presentation of data and statistics.

Of 54 studies of MRI none satisfied more than five of the criteria; 90% of the reports were deficient in eight or more.

It has been suggested that early studies are usually simply descriptive [102] and that once the method is established ways can be developed to produce a statistically acceptable comparison trial. The difficulty with such an approach is that once the machinery is bought and widely distributed it is extremely difficult to put together trial protocols which are not biased towards its continued use. Indeed it might be thought that, even if only minimally effective, such expensive machinery cannot ethically be abandoned.

This is a problem with all costly developments in medicine. At the early stages the approach is not fully developed and therefore the evaluation is likely to be negative. At later stages there is a commitment to the new approach and any evaluation which shows that the method does not work will tend to be ignored. There is also a legal difficulty which is that once a method, whether evaluated or not, is regarded as being part of routine diagnostic treatment by the profession at large, there may be an onus on practitioners to use that method whatever the scientific evidence for its effectiveness on *a priori* grounds.

Effectiveness of scanning: UK examples

A recent study in the UK compared CT and MRI for investigating lesions within the brain in the posterior cranial fossa, normally a very difficult part of the brain to envisage using other methods [103]. Patients were randomly allocated to CT scan or MRI. The doctors in charge of the patients were then asked if they were happy with the diagnosis or if they required the other form of imaging to be carried out.

MRI was very effective at diagnosing abnormal posterior cranial fossae. As proof of this, one in five of those patients who initially had CT scanning were referred for MRI whereas only one in 20 of those who initially had MRI were referred for CT in order to be sure of the diagnosis. It must be said, however, that the main use of both scanning types was to exclude suspected tumours or other disease. In this study therefore the imaging was not helpful in reaching an initial diagnosis, indeed it was used to exclude the suspected diagnosis.

Of those people who did have a disease in the posterior fossa of their brain, CT scanning was satisfactory in 16 and MRI in 19 cases out of 20. MRI was therefore slightly better than CT scanning although the study did not give any information about whether the MRI was cost effective and whether patients improved as a result of treatment for those diseases diagnosed by the imaging process.

In another study [104], 100 patients receiving MRI were compared with another 100 referred for spinal imaging using X-rays. The MRI caused clinicians to change their diagnosis in a fifth of the cases and there was a change in the way that the patient was managed in almost two-thirds of the patients seen. Despite these changes the patient's quality of life was not improved in those who had MRI compared with other patients. As far as patients were concerned there was no advantage in having the costly test.

The Medical Research Council (MRC) [105] undertook a report on the cost effectiveness of MRI which showed that the cost of MRI is much greater than that of CT scanning, largely because far fewer patients can be imaged in a day using MRI. On the other hand, if MRI is compared with an invasive investigation such as myelography, where dye is injected into patients to outline different organs, the costs of going into hospital have to be included and therefore the average costs of MRI and the invasive procedure are very similar. The MRC report also suggested that there was no need to invest in MRI as well as CT scanning except when a hospital is a regional centre.

REDUCING DEPENDENCE ON HOSPITAL: ABDOMINAL DISEASE

High technology can be used to accelerate the move towards community care by reducing the need for inpatient stay in hospital. A particular example that has been explored is gastrointestinal disease [106]. This study concentrated on gastrointestinal endoscopy, an area where medicine, surgery and radiology overlap, so that the move towards community care also involved a blurring of the traditional divisions within medicine.

At present, care and therapy for gastrointestinal diseases are given more or less equally to patients as inpatients or outpatients. In future, it was felt, most will be looked after as day cases. Diagnostic endoscopy in this specialty is now offered by physicians, surgeons and radiologists depending on which area or unit a patient is referred to. This suggests that as these joint units develop there will be a blurring of the tasks that professionals perform.

The authors of the study set up a Delphi exercise in order to reach a consensus about the types of changes likely to occur in the treatment of gastrointestinal disease. In the first instance this consisted of separate interviews with each professional providing services. The second stage involved getting the people together at a meeting to discuss the possible ways that clinical treatment would progress in the future.

An example used by this group will illustrate the way that they work. They gave three possible options for the treatment of duodenal ulcer. In the first case, a general practitioner refers patients directly to a hospital-based consultant who confirms the presence of a duodenal ulcer by endoscopy and monitors the treatment given. In the second case, the general practitioner once again refers to hospital where minimally invasive therapy is carried out. A third approach is totally community based; the general practitioner performs open access endoscopy to confirm the diagnosis and initiates and monitors therapy.

All three approaches were considered to be satisfactory in terms of their safety and acceptability by the experts. They felt that the community approach was the most efficient and cost effective. In addition, it was felt that it was marginally safer, largely because of a reduced chance of cross-infection. It was felt that most patients would prefer the community based route, though it was suggested that for first attacks of duodenal ulcer symptoms most patients would prefer no investigation. It was felt that in the future all patients with uncomplicated duodenal ulcer would be treated in the community. This may require some slightly extended general practitioner training but the use of hospital services will be restricted only to those patients who have poor initial results.

This sort of exercise was used for a number of different gastrointestinal diseases in this study. These included endoscopy, duodenal ulcer, treatment of gall stones and cancer of the colon and rectum. Apart from cancer of the colon and rectum the experts felt that all of these problems would, in the not too distant future, largely be cared for in the community.

The study then looked at the likely effect on the use of hospitals as a result of these suggested changes and the more general effects on the demand for care, such as the ageing of the population and other demographic changes. They put forward the possibility that smaller hospitals, perhaps staffed by specialists visiting from larger sites or local staff with special training, would form the central point of newly designed diagnostic centres. These are much commoner in other countries than in the UK, though there is a move to reestablish small hospitals in some localities in the UK.

There will need to be an improvement in the training of general practitioners if they are to take on the development of therapy in such centres. The British tradition, however, has been in a different direction, with the specialists providing secondary care moving out into the community, either entirely or with part of their practice remaining in a hospital setting. There is already evidence within the UK of general practitioner fundholders showing interest in hospital consultants providing services in their immediate locality rather than having their patients travel to a central point. The recent reorganization of the health service has therefore once again tended to cause a dispersal of expertise traditionally held in hospital settings. Another possibility is that the equipment could be mounted in vehicles and taken to different places requiring the service.

The most interesting conclusion of this set of studies was that medical practitioners were capable of taking on greater responsibilities and that they would give greater benefit both to patients and to the service in general by doing so. The general practitioner would be more involved in identifying what the patient needs, explaining what the options were and preparing the way for whatever intervention might be undertaken. It seems likely that the general practitioners will, in turn, move much of their present workload onto other members of the primary care team. It has been shown that nurse practitioners can undertake much of the general practitioner's routine work. With a good screening process, the primary care nurse can also be of great assistance in taking over some of the general practitioner's workload.

TECHNOLOGIES WHICH WILL ENHANCE HOME CARE

Several advances in technology have been taken up by the medical professions for the development of home and community based care. Developments in office and management methods are as useful to the health service as to any manufacturing company. Telecommunications and computer technology are good examples of this. Many of the new technologies will help with the development of a less institutionalized health service [107]. Technological developments for people living at home have been emerging over the last few years. Sometimes they are obviously effective, but there needs to be as much scrutiny of these as of any other new approach. Some of the technologies that will lessen the need for inpatient services over the next decade or so are:

- diagnostic kits and desk top analysers
- assessment systems using personal computers
- new vaccines
- laparoscopy and endoscopy
- vascular catheters with or without lasers
- laser microsurgery and vaporization (e.g. for tumours)
- computer controlled prostheses
- treatment and drug delivery systems.

The development of monoclonal antibodies will be especially useful in reducing the need for inpatient care. These antibodies are substances produced from the culture of living tissues. They have a very long life and are produced by fusing together an antibody-forming white cell, known as a lymphocyte, with a tumour cell often derived from mouse myeloma cells [108]. The antibody can be made specifically to react with a particular protein and can therefore be made to seek out abnormal cells. They link with suspicious cells in the body of a patient and help to identify what problem the patient is suffering from, and in future they may even be used to destroy the abnormal cells. The antibodies, if they contain small amounts of radioactive material, can be detected and used for outlining abnormal tissues without surgery. Abnormal cells (e.g. cancer cells or blood vessels which are blocked) can be traced using this method. The tests can give diagnostic information quickly and may allow patients to remain at home or to have a shorter stay in hospital.

Diagnostic kits can be used in clinics or at home with little expertise on the part of the person using them. The commonest uses for such kits at present are for diagnosing pregnancy or ovulation, with the kit being used to detect the presence of certain hormones. They can also be used for deciding on the cause of respiratory infections, and the presence of some bacteria, such as streptococci, and sexually transmitted diseases.

Tests for a number of diseases may eventually be offered on sale to the public, including screening tests for cancer of the cervix or prostate. A wide variety of other kits may be used to diagnose skin diseases, tooth decay and eye problems. Some companies plan to develop and market tests for common diseases with a partly genetic cause, such as diabetes [109]. The kits, together with new analysers, allow reliable diagnostic testing virtually anywhere. A high proportion of patients admitted to hospital at present are there to have their diagnosis confirmed, treatment often being possible at home.

New developments in immunology have also opened up the field of vaccination. Firstly, improvements in present day vaccines can reduce side-effects. An example of a vaccine that may be improved by new methods is the influenza vaccine. This should cause a marked reduction in the development of pandemics, which have spread throughout the world in the past. Some other effective vaccines have been developed recently including one against *Haemophilus* meningitis.

Other aspects of technology: self care

Technology, especially in the media and communications industries, can provide more interactive ways of curing, caring and training. This includes the possibility of patients interrogating, from their own homes, either a suitably programmed machine or an expert in the problem that they have and to receive therapy for it. At first sight such an approach appears far fetched, but virtually all the technological problems have been solved. It is simply a matter of acceptability. The concern is that such methods will simply maintain the existing obsessions.

It is not the place of this book to delve into the collective unconscious to try to find out why humans, in developed countries at any rate, prefer to rely on machines or strangers than people they know. For example, we queue outside bank machines rather than face the tellers inside the bank or buy clothes in self-service shops rather than have a clothes assistant providing a personal service. In medicine, young people prefer to get contraceptive advice from clinics staffed by people they do not know, or condoms from machines, rather than from their general practitioner. They are willing to rely on machines for medical help.

New advances need to be approached with three basic questions: 'Does it do something useful?'; if so 'Does it do it better than the best alternative?'; if so 'Is the advantage such that it will not deprive anyone else of effective treatment?', which usually involves its being reasonably cheap. If the answers to these questions are all 'yes', technological changes can result in improved methods of prevention, diagnosis and treatment of disease. The changes that are discernible will certainly allow us to redefine the need for and place of hospitals in the health service. The reason for this is that with some of the new technological changes much of the cure and care given by health services will be possible in the patient's home or in small units, such as the general practitioner's surgery, away from hospitals [110].

I have mentioned that advances in communications and the development of self-contained packages for prevention, diagnosis, treatment and rehabilitation will allow a move from centralized facilities. This will have the advantage of making the bulk of the services currently provided in hospital more accessible. It will also allow patients to have considerable influence on the way services are provided and developed.

It seems likely that a few very specialized, surgical procedures will be provided in small intensive care units, but that these will back up the main, community based activities. These intensive procedures will probably include transplantation surgery and, initially at least, some genetic manipulations, more because of the need for close access to multidisciplinary teams and facilities than because of patient needs.

Allowing disabled people to stay at home

A number of new technological developments assist people who would normally depend on their family or their health providers. Treatments include artificial sphincters and electrical stimulators for the prevention of urinary incontinence to relieve problems caused by poor bladder function. In future, an aim will be to develop devices that replace parts of the nervous system. These stimulate nerve fibres or nerve cells electrically and restore functions that have been lost because of disease or injury. One type of device that has recently been in the news is the use of cochleal implants to improve hearing. Other devices are likely to follow for speech and even smell [111–113].

These devices work by electrically stimulating nerves, parts of the spinal cord, or areas within the brain, in an attempt to simulate the normal signals given off by those organs and improve senses that are damaged. The aim of these advances is to make dependent people more independent and to keep them out of hospitals and other institutions.

Other developments include a number of new methods for continuously delivering drugs. The idea of these, in some cases, is to avoid the variations in blood level at different times that are likely with intermittent injections [114]. Such pumps and subcutaneous reservoirs will find more and more uses in future. Some pumps can react to the needs of the patient by altering the dose. People with diabetes and those needing chemical treatment of cancer or those with blood clotting problems are already using these methods. Continuous morphine can be infused in people with chronic pain. Many of these drug delivery systems will allow people with chronic illness to lead more independent lives away from institutions.

Some approaches to new technology tackle the surroundings of disabled people. Controls can be used to allow people to manipulate the doors and windows to their homes, and the electrical apparatus, lighting and heating, and to assist with mobility up and down stairs within the home. These ideas will expand with the development of robotics for undertaking household and other tasks. At the very basic end new aids for helping with lifting patients have made it possible for people to be cared for at home where previously that would have been impossible because of a lack of manpower.

Not all new technologies allow us to substitute central, hospital-based services for more peripheral ones. Some (e.g. intensive care and organ transplantation) require complex facilities near at hand and the immediate availability of teams of highly skilled people. Some of this work may be better performed using mobile emergency facilities, along the lines of the more successful coronary care units, but some will probably have to remain in a central place [115].

OTHER APPROACHES

Simpler approaches to surgery, for instance in draining abscesses in diverticular disease, have been made possible by the use of ultrasound scanning. A fine tube can be inserted through the skin into such abscesses under ultrasound scanning control, which allows the therapy to be performed without anaesthetic or major operation [116]. The effect of such changes on the use of hospitals will be considerable because it will mean that patients will have only minimal discomfort under local anaesthetic. This will not require the complex theatre suites which have grown up in hospital. Indeed much of the treatment can be given from a general practitioner's premises.

Further developments in diagnosis will be brought about by the use of fibre optics. The method allows images to be passed along narrow flexible tubes, allowing the specialist to visualize directly virtually every part of the body. In addition, endoscopes will be able to incorporate tiny cameras and pass images back from those cameras in digitalized form. The ability to image any part of the body can be added to by the provision of a cutting and cauterizing ability in the form of miniature lasers. These are increasingly used in surgical treatments for destroying unhealthy or abnormal tissue. Lasers are well established in surgery of the eye and skin. In eye surgery, lasers are used to treat eye changes in diabetics [117]. Lasers are still to be evaluated in a number of other treatments including the cauterization of upper gastrointestinal bleeding and treatment of early cancer of the cervix of the uterus.

In future, it may be possible to use coloured lasers with coloured antibodies to destroy specified tissues, possibly cancerous tumours. The abnormal cells will be used to produce specific antibodies which will be coloured. When these are injected the abnormal tissues will take up the cells and the colour. In theory this will allow relatively untrained staff to use coloured lasers to destroy tissues of the same colour (and therefore abnormal), without affecting the normal surrounding organs. The laser will seal off any bleeding and will be capable of passing through normal tissue, including the skin, without harm. This obviously has great implications for surgical practice where abnormal cells need to be destroyed, allowing much of that work to be carried out at home or in the general practitioner's surgery by the district nurse.

Lasers, used with endoscopes or catheters, can reach many parts of the body through the gut, the air passages and the urinary tract. Lasers carried by catheters in the arteries can be carried to the coronary arteries and used to destroy clots or thrombi. They have the benefit of removing blockages, while at the same time smoothing the vessel wall which may have been blocked [118].

5	# Pressures for change: consumer choice

IMPORTANCE OF CONSUMERS HAVING A CHOICE

It may at first seem obvious that patients, as consumers of health care, should have some choice in the type of care they receive, as far as best practice will allow, and that they should be satisfied with the choice of care they make. Making such an approach central to the organization of the health service is quite new to the UK, where the tradition has long been that the professionals know best. Since the development of the purchaser and provider system, purchasers have had a duty to discover what makes the different parts of the health service satisfactory or unsatisfactory from the patient's point of view. As a result, surveys measuring patients' satisfaction with the health service in the UK have greatly increased in number [119, 120]. Giving patients a choice at the point of delivery of the service is still unusual.

The views of patients on the different services and their satisfaction with one approach as contrasted with another are important, but there are traps for the unwary, even for this rather superficial exercise. There is little point in asking someone's view of the their residential home if they know that they have no option but to stay there. Likewise, to ask a woman with breast cancer if she would rather have her breast removed or have only the lump removed without a full explanation of why there is a choice at all, is pointless when her main concern is survival. If both are truly equally safe there is no option, the less mutilating the operation the better. Giving patients the option in that circumstance simply opens the way for those choosing the lesser operation to feel extreme guilt if the operation fails.

Nevertheless, one of the most powerful ways of deciding whether the quality of health services is reasonable is to ask the patients who have been treated by that service how it affected them [121]. This is not simply because of a desire to please, or to boost the reputation of a service and therefore the people providing it. Some authors [122, 123] have suggested that patient satisfaction is important because satisfied patients are more likely to cooperate with the people giving them their health care. They are more likely to fulfil their part of the implied bargain which is struck whenever patients meet doctors. For example, they will take whatever medication or advice they have been given. However, there are problems with looking at patient satisfaction as a way of helping with the planning of services.

Service knowledge

The first of these is that some patients, if they have not already received the service, or were not clear about its nature when they received it, remain unaware of its existence. This was found to be the case when questioning people about services, especially some community services [124]. The study examined the attitudes of 250 people on the general practitioners' registers in Cardiff. They were aged 75 years and over and were asked about services they were likely to receive, or had already received. Figure 5.1 shows that a high proportion of these people were unaware of the existence or function of some of the services provided by health and social services in Cardiff.

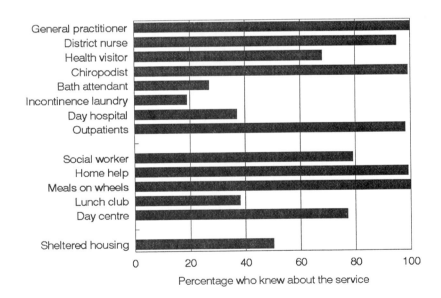

Figure 5.1 Percentage of elderly people who knew of the existence of services.

A number of other studies have found relatively low levels of awareness of different health and social services among samples of people [125]. Other authors have shown that levels of demand for services are altered by the health and disability of the recipients of the service. They are also altered by patients' knowledge of, and willingness to use, services and by the reputation of that service [126].

Service satisfaction

Connelly and Goldberg, reviewing attitudes to a particular service (meals on wheels), reported that most studies about the service show that people receiving it reveal a 'high degree of satisfaction' [127]. However, the reviewers comment that it is difficult to know whether real opinions are being given. Some people may fear withdrawal of the existing services or do not want to appear ungrateful. This may bias the response given by people, especially if they are a group who believe that they may need the service at some future time. Even worse, they may be under the care of such a service at the time of the interview.

Several studies have shown that older clients report themselves more satisfied with services than those in younger age groups. Connelly and Goldberg observed that researchers in this field have been cautious of accepting stated views at face value since 'this generation of old people are likely to have low expectations and lack of knowledge of alternatives'. They also note that, despite a high level of expressed general satisfaction, a lot of people taking part in consumer studies had specific complaints when directly questioned. Much appears to depend on the way in which questions are asked [128] and the amount of detail asked for.

Attitudes to institutions

A recent study in Hackney, east London, found that fewer than half of the people on the waiting list for residential care were 'looking forward' to entering an institution, and a quarter stated spontaneously that they had no wish to go [129]. The study showed that the main advantages of residential care were thought to be 'companionship' and 'being looked after'. The most frequently quoted disadvantage was 'loss of independence'.

A study of public preferences for care in Scotland, found widespread antipathy to institutional care, an emotion which was most strongly associated with geriatric hospitals [130]. This antagonism was found no matter how ill the people asked and did not change according to age or whether people lived alone. People who had been in a geriatric ward or hospital had more animosity towards going in again than the general public who had not visited one [131], so it did not appear to be a fear of the unknown that prompted such sentiments. The difference in attitude between those who have been treated by a ward or other service and those who have not is a useful way of measuring the reputation of a particular place or service and whether this appears to be deserved.

Kennedy and Acland found that most patients regarded admission to hospital as likely to be a permanent move; 'over and over again, it was made clear that elderly people thought of hospital chiefly as a place to die'. The dislike of the place expressed by patients revolved around complaints about restrictions imposed by hospital routine, noise and lack of cigarettes [132].

A more recent study, designed to investigate attitudes and fears of elderly lucid patients about admission to a geriatric unit, found that about a quarter of the patients were distressed by the presence of confused patients. Those in the higher social classes reacted significantly more unfavourably than those in the lower [133]. Many of these patients became distressed when the topic of residential home admission was discussed. Only a third said they would have no anxieties about admission and four out of 10 could think of no advantages at all. The main problem identified by the study was of losing independence, the main gain that of being looked after. The poor state of the other patients in geriatric wards is often cited as their worst aspect.

CHOICES FOR PEOPLE TO BE ADMITTED

It is an astonishing fact, given the cost of hospital admission, that where researchers have measured the need for admission against standard criteria, the majority of people going into hospital did not need to go in. Indeed their admission and stay has, more often than not, been shown to be not just unnecessary but inappropriate. The criteria used in theses studies have not assumed that new services are available, or that any change needs to take place to accommodate these people elsewhere. The criteria are usually drawn up by the clinicians running the local services in their existing state. These findings are discussed in more detail in Chapter 6.

A number of studies have compared the attitudes of patients to services in different settings. The most relevant to this book compared hospital based and non-hospital based care. A study of particular interest looked at day surgery based in a large teaching hospital [134] in the suburbs of a city in northern California. This was compared with a free-standing surgical unit. This approach is interesting because it shows that surgery can be undertaken outside what would normally be defined as a hospital. The facility, which was attached to a large general practice, consisted of an operating room, a three-bed recovery unit, a minor procedures room, waiting and reception areas and a patient changing room.

In order to compare their degree of satisfaction, patients were restricted to those who had had one particular procedure – a cataract extraction. Ninety-eight patients had been to the free-standing day hospital and 95 had been to the hospital based day hospital. The effectiveness of the procedures, measured in terms of the physical and mental state of patients, was similar for both groups and therefore the study revolved around the preference of the patients for one or other of the day units. The groups were not randomized but the patients appeared to be very similar in terms of age, sex and severity of the disease before being treated.

There was no difference in the degree of satisfaction with technical aspects of the care, namely the way that the operation seemed to be performed, the personal relationships with staff and the degree to which patients trusted the staff, when measured on standardized scales between the two groups (Figure 5.2). It is interesting that the free-standing day unit scored lower (i.e. better) on all scores but this difference was not great enough to rule out a chance finding.

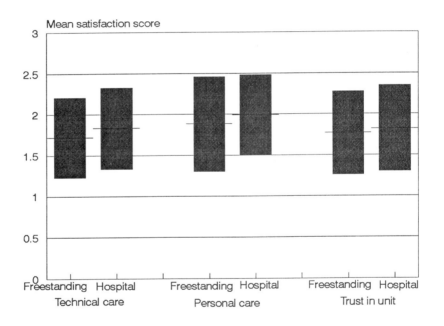

Figure 5.2 Patients using free-standing or hospital day surgery were equally satisfied with technical competence. Mean score (horizontal line); plus or minus standard deviation (vertical line).

However, when less technical aspects were examined, especially the comfort of the surroundings, the convenience of getting to the unit, the courtesy of staff and the speed and seriousness with which complaints were handled, the free-standing day hospital scored much better and the patients treated there were thus significantly more satisfied (Figure 5.3).

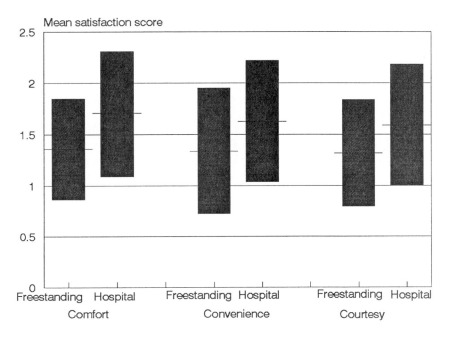

Figure 5.3 Patients using free-standing surgery were more satisfied with comfort, convenience and courtesy than those using hospital day surgery. Mean score (horizontal line); plus or minus standard deviation (vertical line).

In particular, and perhaps not surprisingly, patients were more satisfied with the ease and convenience of getting to the free-standing local day unit. There was also a marked difference in the amount of courtesy and consideration shown by receptionists and secretaries in the free-standing unit, though there was no difference in the satisfaction patients felt with the work of the physicians or nurses.

This was quite a small study and was not methodologically entirely satisfactory. It was not, for instance, a randomized trial, which means that it is possible that the patients going to one facility or the other had important differences in their attitudes to care before they went into the day hospitals. However, the study did show, over a range of measures, that good results can be obtained for day surgery in units that are peripherally based, rather than being in a central hospital complex, and that these appear to be preferred by patients.

REMOVING BUILDINGS: MENTAL ILLNESS SERVICES

Patients are part of wider society, so that when they state preferences their choices are difficult to disentangle from attitudes set by society at large, possibly as part of a fashion or fad, or part of a political or social movement. These preferences are, in turn, often difficult to disentangle from political actions. These may hold and press opinions on what is best for people who are unwell, as a result of a much broader aim, not necessarily directly related to the well-being of patients.

A good example of changes that are supposed to increase choices for patients is seen in those to the mental illness services. A move away from hospital towards community care has, at least partially, resulted from a broader political movement, originating in the civil rights movement in the USA. Mentally ill people must have been affected by the pressure of such groups which have been vociferous in suggesting that mentally ill people are disadvantaged rather than being ill, or are at least made worse because of the way they are treated. The difficulty with policies based on fashion, even if, as I believe, they are ultimately correct, is twofold. The policy tends to get pushed forward faster than is reasonable for the patients or the development of the new alternative service, so that people may be moved from hospital before community services are fully developed. Also, policy based on fashion may swing back, influenced by singular and spectacular failures of that policy, again to the great detriment of patients.

The move towards community care for mentally ill people has a long history. In part it reflects therapeutic advances, but it also represents a change in emphasis on the way that mentally ill people should be thought of, the policy of normalization. This developed from a number of sources. Some psychiatrists in the USA initiated an open door policy for mentally ill people in the 1950s [135]. This was followed by the civil rights campaigns of the 1960s suggesting that putting mentally ill people in mental institutions was a form of discrimination, causing, rather than alleviating their condition. Other changes in society about that time resulted in a loss of confidence in experts. This was especially noticeable in the USA where the loss of confidence in doctors was triggered partly by their acquisition of great wealth and partly by the spectacular damages awarded against those who were sued, suggesting that they were not all-knowing.

A rise in the status of sociology theory and social work as a profession, plus a holistic approach to care rather than a mechanistic one, all played their part in putting pressure on the move towards community based social care rather than hospital based treatment. A further, less altruistic, element was a general belief and a little initial evidence [136] that community based care can prove less costly, at least in terms of the costs which would have to be met by the government. The low status of psychiatry within the medical profession and its relative isolation from the rest of the medical establishment, often literally so in large rural hospitals, meant that its power bases were not heavily defended by the profession at large.

This process was widespread, but the UK was not particularly in the forefront of moves towards caring for more severely mentally ill people in the community. Large scale schemes were introduced in the USA and then in Italy, with The Netherlands, Australia and New Zealand all making policy moves in the same direction. The UK followed a policy of gradualism, probably for the usual reason in the UK, that no one would pay for rapid change. This meant that some areas moved quickly towards a community based mental illness service, others more slowly, others hardly at all.

There is no real evidence that these changes were initiated as a result of patient dissatisfaction or pressure from relatives of people with mental illness. Indeed some relatives' groups remain implacably opposed to the development of community care for mentally ill people because of the fear that they will be abandoned to look after demanding and socially embarrassing people in their own homes.

What evidence there is about the views of mentally ill people themselves suggests that the new approach does seem to be preferred where it has been implemented well [137]. Patients who have been in hospital for many years have been shown to be able to use shops and pubs, to have fewer behaviour problems, improved morale and better skills.

The mental illness services have had more experience of moving patients from hospital into the community than virtually any other service, but it is still rare for patients to be asked how they feel about the move. It is perceived as being difficult to know how to measure the satisfaction of patients, especially long stay patients, with services [138]. A number of patients have known little else but inpatient care and are naturally reluctant to change. Thus, some recent work in this field on the change over from hospital to community based psychiatric care has suggested that patients are generally satisfied with the institutions they are using [139].

I have already mentioned some of the general difficulties of trying to ask patients, especially those who are vulnerable, about their satisfaction. Mentally ill people may give answers that are ambiguous [140, 141] so that high satisfaction or low satisfaction scores may be of questionable value.

A number of authors have studied the change from a hospital to community based service [142]. It is curious that of all the patient subgroups, those who have been in mental illness institutions for some time or those who have depended heavily on such institutions intermittently over a period, should be the group that is expected to move into community care first. It seems likely that of all the patients within the health care service this group will find the move the most difficult. On the other hand, it does suggest that if we can implement this reasonably well and humanely the rest will be easy.

There is no point in asking patients to compare two services where one of them is substandard. Given such a dependent group it is not surprising that at least half of the patients questioned in different surveys tend to be satisfied no matter what service is under scrutiny. In a useful overview of studies looking at consumer satisfaction, Corrigan [143] looked in more detail at why patients were satisfied, whether it was to do with the quality of staff relationships, the surroundings, or the degree of freedom and the amount of information that patients have about their disease and their medication.

The overview showed some differences in attitude. For instance Corrigan quotes McEvoy and colleagues in 1981 [144] who found that only 40% of a sample of mentally ill people had any idea of what was wrong with them and about half of them believed that their medication was unnecessary. This was not particularly related to the insight that the patient was capable of with regard to his or her disease; the degree of ignorance was not part of the disease process. A number of workers have shown that patients' attitudes about their quality of care in both inpatient and community settings fit reasonably well with 'reality', in other words, their views correlate closely with the impressions of treatment staff [145, 146].

Attitudes of mentally ill people to hospitals

Patients' attitudes towards their therapy in general were mixed. Some authors found that this stemmed in part from patients being unhappy with a lack of information about the likely effects of medicines. Some studies found that, for instance, group therapy was not liked. Patients were particularly keen to have free time for recreational activities. Most patients were highly dissatisfied with any seclusion as inpatients and a number felt that it was used as a punishment rather than for their safety. In terms of the physical characteristics of inpatient care, a lack of privacy was most important.

A central complaint about the staffing of the hospitals was about the rigid hierarchy, with those at the top making all of the important decisions, but not being easy to contact, while those at the bottom were unable to make decisions. There was also a fixed distinction between managerial staff and the decisions they were able to make and clinical staff and the decisions that fell under their jurisdiction at the top. This caste system often caused considerable disadvantage to patients, especially with regard to changes in treatment regimes and preparations that needed to be made for discharge from the hospital. Such hierarchies may impinge most obviously on mentally ill patients, especially those held in hospital against their will, but the same rigid approach is an inherent attribute of most hospitals (Figure 5.4) [147].

The rigid structure is not the only way of organizing hospital life, but it is found so commonly that one suspects that the easiest way of altering it may be to move away from hospital care into the community. A number of authors have suggested that with proper preparation, discharge can be seen by most patients as the ultimate success.

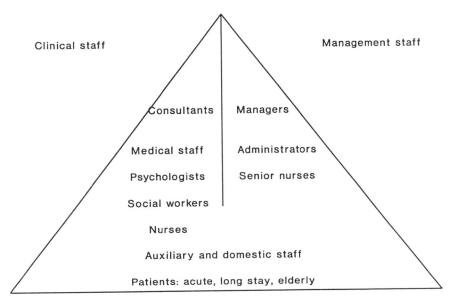

Figure 5.4 The hospital hierarchy. (Reproduced with permission from [147].)

Mentally ill patients in general hospitals

Acutely mentally ill people are increasingly being managed, during the acute phase of their illness, away from mental illness hospitals in district general hospitals. This is said to be less stigmatizing and allows psychiatrists and other professionals in the mental illness field to be in contact with the rest of the inpatient orientated health professionals. It seems to me that this is likely to be a halfway phase while we decide on what it is that hospitals do best.

There is good evidence that much of the acute care given to mentally ill people can be provided with advantage in their own homes. This is described in more detail in Chapter 7. Those who do need close 24-hour attention are likely to be managed, as in my own area, in self-contained units set up in small towns or city suburbs.

The closure of mental illness hospitals and their replacement by small acute, preferably local and homely, units is no longer an issue in most areas of the UK today. The decisions and plans have been made. We do need care, compassion, some imagination and some cash to implement them, but the battles are over.

PATIENT CHOICE: THE EXAMPLE OF CHILDREN

The development of home care services for children has been an important move towards giving parents and children more choice in the way they should be cared for. Research has shown that some of the effects on children of being taken into hospital can be quite damaging [148, 149], particularly for those under 5 years of age and admitted on a number of occasions [150]. Despite this, the development of alternatives to hospital has been slow. This appears to have been because of the problem, which will by now be increasingly familiar to the reader, of an excessive belief in the importance of high technology and the attendant belief that this can only be provided in hospital.

There also appears to be a problem of perception. There is a tradition that specialists give care in hospitals and that for them to stray outside the walls, apart from occasional brief visits, is costly and in some way lowers their status. There are no studies to show the former and a few honourable exceptions disprove the latter. It is now generally accepted that home care is a particularly attractive option for young children. Apart from avoiding the consequences of their going into hospital, they usually have parents or other relatives available who are expert at caring for their day-to-day needs and who can, with a little extra training, oversee their care. For children, a particularly important physical consequence of not going to hospital is that they avoid hospital acquired infection.

It has been shown that parents are capable of performing complicated tasks [151] and parental involvement reduces anxiety both in parents and in the children [152]. The Department of Health has made it clear that parents should now have a voice in choosing where children should be cared for [153].

A small study [154] has shown that although the majority of parents are reasonably satisfied with their experience in hospital, a minority have strong feelings about the need to improve care. A particular theme identified by people who had been in hospital as being extremely important, was a lack of information. A number of parents also made comments about the lack of discharge planning. A few children were discharged with virtually no notice.

Parents were expected to take part in assisting with care of children in hospital and although they were all pleased that this should be the case, felt that their other commitments, particularly other children at home were ignored by hospital staff. Virtually all of the parents questioned who had experienced both types of care expressed a preference for home rather than hospital care. They regarded their children as being more relaxed at home, happier and more comfortable. Family unity was better preserved despite the strains that an ill child imposed on it. It was remarked that the food was much better at home than in hospital. The facilities for parents were not particularly good in many of the hospitals looked at.

The visiting teams giving home care were found to be much more forthcoming as far as information was concerned. The staff involved seemed to feel that it was their task to keep parents informed. Staff were willing to give time to talk through problems that were likely to occur and answer questions. It is curious that staff felt better able to give information to parents at home than in hospital. The home care staff appeared to be much keener to teach parents to undertake the different processes that were needed for children treated at home and while doing this would explain why they needed to be done. Parents made the point that home care was much less costly to them than hospital care in terms of time, travelling and queuing. This has been noted by a number of previous researchers [155–157].

A good example of paediatric community care has been set up in Nottingham where half of all paediatric surgical operations are done on a day case basis. This is thought to speed up recovery and the children feel more comfortable at home. There are 17 specialist nurses including six paediatric community nurses based in the hospital. These paediatric community nurses work with the families and liaise with the general practitioners and health visitors in the local general practices.

There are also nurses who specialize in particular conditions such as diabetes, cystic fibrosis and asthma. The emphasis is on giving advice to parents in the home if there is any difficulty or any complications of the treatment. The emphasis on communication with the general practitioners in primary care has meant that children can be discharged sooner because of the increased skills which the primary care team has gained from access to the specialists. Parents have been given advice on how to help children directly with complex problems, such as the management of tracheostomies. An important part of the service is that parents can phone up the nurses at any time to get advice if difficulties arise.

Another idea that has been developed has been the community care of children who have bony injuries as a result of trauma. The county also has two nurses who specialize in the treatment of cancer patients in the community. One ensures that information about the complex therapy required, such as chemotherapy, blood transfusions or investigation, is available while the other ensures that families are fully informed about the therapy. The nurses specializing in asthma spend time explaining to parents and school staff the complexities of caring for a child who has asthma.

VARIATIONS IN THE SERVICE PROVIDED BY HOSPITALS

The NHS and Community Care Act has highlighted some information that was available but which had been ignored for some time. This centres round the great variation in the use of hospitals for what appears to be the same disease in different places, suggesting that there is a great deal of waste in the system as it stands. Some American figures have suggested that in the treatment of children there are 18-fold differences in the rate of admission to hospital for gastroenteritis and 15-fold differences for respiratory disease [158]. Wennberg and Kim have shown sixfold differences for bronchitis and fivefold differences for pneumonia [159].

A study comparing only teaching hospitals showed fivefold differences for respiratory tract infection [160]. The risks of being admitted to hospital for surgical conditions were also markedly different. It may be argued that these differences are simply due to some areas of the country having more sickness than others. However, in three diagnoses (bacterial meningitis, fracture of the femur and appendicitis) which are very specific, severe diagnoses that can be verified, the rates of hospitalization were very similar, suggesting that where there are more objective descriptions of a disease the admission policy varies less. It also suggests that for less precise, less severe conditions, admission policies vary greatly in their approach, some of which must be extremely wasteful of resources [161].

ARE GOVERNMENTS DEVELOPING CHEAPER OPTIONS?

A number of UK government documents have promoted community care over the last 20 years or so, culminating in the community care aspects of the Community Care Act. The information I give in this book appears to show that community care is usually cheaper than home care if only those costs which have to be met by the health service are taken into account. If costs to others, especially the costs to the family in terms of lost wages and commitment to the patient, are taken into account the costs appear to be roughly equivalent or a little cheaper, depending on the type of patient, the degree of dependency and the availability of family members [162].

There is therefore a danger that, in order to make community care cheaper, support for carers may not be as intensive as it has been in the early, successful experiments. There is a feeling in some professional circles that such neglect will not be noticed. There is a reasonable hypothesis which suggests that the opposite is true; that neglect in hospital is easier to get away with. The reason for this is that home care is more accessible to families and the public generally so that poor care is noticed. It is true that there are occasions where this has not been the case. Old people have been found dead in their homes days or even months after death, but I would submit that these cases hit the headlines because they are unusual. It is my experience that such neglect is likely to occur and, perhaps worse, to be tolerated in closed communities, whether hospitals, residential or nursing homes, without being remarked on [163]. The development of geriatrics as a specialty was partly accelerated by the previous acceptance in the UK of such neglect in the old local authority hospitals [164].

PEOPLE'S PREFERENCES: IS HOME CARE DANGEROUS?

The pressure from consumers to have home care where there is an option is difficult to oppose as a growing amount of evidence suggests that there is little done in hospital that cannot be better done at home. The evidence is not even particularly new. There is, however, a marked inclination, especially in the professions, to resist the move. Many of the trials and experiments made to compare home with hospital therapy have struck a degree of obstruction which is almost unsurpassed since 'teaching against Galen' stopped being a crime.

More and more diseases can be treated with shorter hospital stays than has previously been the case. For some conditions there is doubt about the need for hospital admission at all. A number of scientific trials have tested whether or not hospital care is effective. They have often been undermined by a lack of support from the local professionals, but a number do suggest either that home care is not dangerous or that it is safer than the hospital equivalent.

A good example was an experiment to test whether home care was as effective as hospital admission for patients with heart attacks. A trial carried out in Bristol [165] showed that people treated in coronary care units in hospital were at a disadvantage compared with those treated at home. Moderately severe cases, which formed the great majority, were more likely to survive at home than those treated in hospital (Figure 5.5). For severe cases there was a slightly higher proportion of deaths for those treated at home. The overall figures were in favour of the group treated at home.

Mather and his colleagues, who set up this study, had considerable difficulty in persuading consultants to take part because just doing the study was considered unethical. Archie Cochrane, the first President of the Faculty of Public Health Medicine, used to describe how he showed the early results of the trial to a number of consultant cardiologists at a meeting. On seeing the results the cardiologists said that, because there was a difference in the death rate the treatment of people at home was unethical and therefore the trial should be discontinued. Cochrane would then move his hand, which until then had hidden the headings above the data, to reveal that the higher death rate was in fact for those treated in hospital. He then suggested that as the difference in mortality rate was enough to be considered unethical all coronary care units should be closed forthwith. This advice was not taken, the main result of this manoeuvre being that a number of consultants became very careful when talking to Cochrane.

The study had some serious drawbacks, largely due to the reluctance of hospital consultants to believe that the study should be undertaken. It was therefore some years before another study was carried out, in Nottingham, where a mobile hospital-based team was called to the homes of patients with symptoms suggestive of coronary heart disease. The mobile team made a decision about whether patients should remain at home or go into hospital, again based on random numbers to prevent preferential treatment or other biases. Three-quarters of the patients visited by the mobile team were included in the

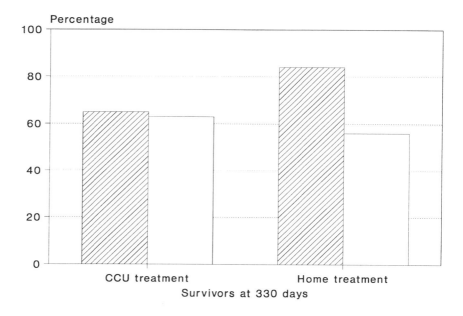

Figure 5.5 Home services showed better survival than hospital (CCU) for moderate cases (shaded); slightly worse for severe cases (unshaded).

study, in contrast to the study in Bristol where only a quarter were allowed to take part.

Once again there was no clear difference between patients treated at home or in hospital. In Nottingham it was suggested that with careful training of general practitioners and with the provision of some high tech equipment, especially cardio-monitors and defibrillators, the whole intensive cardiac service could be transferred to home care with considerable advantages for the patient.

Two main problems appeared to block the continued development of the service in Nottingham. The first was the reluctance of general practitioners to change their methods of working. Patients seen very early on, that is within an hour or two of the onset of the symptoms, were later found to benefit from treatment given to limit the extent of the damage to their heart. This is being used as a reason for the continuation of coronary care units, though the treatment could be better given at home using the Nottingham approach, for the earlier it is given the more effective it is. For people first seen several hours after the onset of their symptoms, treatment entirely at home by skilled personnel, be they general practitioners or others, with a defibrillator at hand would be best.

Coronary heart disease is the commonest single disease in developed countries at this time. People get strokes almost as commonly and they are an important cause of disability in those who suffer them. They also cause a large number of deaths each year. There is no evidence that hospitals have more to offer than home care for preventing the early deaths from stroke. There has been a suggestion that specialist stroke units may be more effective than general hospital wards in preventing early deaths from stroke, though the benefit was lost within a year [166]. This useful meta-analysis includes a number of very different stroke units, with some studies in which mortality was not a primary measure. The main question, as to whether patients might be better off at home has still to be answered for mortality.

The main reason for admitting the majority of stroke cases to hospital at present is to provide rehabilitation therapy. A controlled trial was set up to decide whether admitting people to hospital for the treatment of stroke was useful. Like the Mather study this was carried out in Bristol. People cared for at home received a home care service in addition to the existing community help. The new home service was intended to be used instead of admission to hospital and also to encourage shorter stays for those who were admitted to hospital. The home care team consisted of a nurse, a physiotherapist and a speech therapist. The medical input was provided by the general practitioner.

Once again this trial was not well received by hospital staff. Possibly because of this, the results were confusing [167]. Patients who had the home care team available to them actually spent longer in hospital than the others. Both groups of patients showed very similar rates of deaths and disability, so the difference in therapy made no difference to their rate of progress. The study did show, once again, the difficulty of providing home care services when the hospital service is antagonistic to it and when general practitioners are not sufficiently trained to be able to make full use of the service. What also seems to shine through is that patients treated for acute diseases appear to be as well off at home as in hospital as long as some very basic facilities are available.

A less controversial approach has been to try to reduce the length of stay in hospital of people with acute diseases or to shorten the length of their treatment for long term problems. Virtually all of these have shown that there is no difference in the well-being of patients between those treated for a short period and those for what was, at the time, the standard length of therapy.

One of the earlier trials spotlighted hernias and varicose veins [168]. This showed no disadvantage in terms of complications to patients discharged earlier, nor did they appear to require much extra further support.

A trial which looked at 11 surgical and two medical categories was carried out in Canada [169]. Despite careful preparation of the patients, a high proportion of those who should have been treated at home were in fact sent into hospital. In five of the conditions, home care proved to be more cost effective than hospital care largely because of the reduction in the length of stay. There was no difference in any of the measures of patient well-being, including their psychological state and their ability to get back to work. There appeared to be little economic benefit for home care in this study, but it was some years ago (1976).

THE SPECIAL CASE OF MATERNITY SERVICES

Counter to the trend in other acute specialties, maternity services have been increasing the proportion of patients who deliver their babies in hospital over the past 20 years, though lengths of stay have decreased. This appears to have been against the wishes of many mothers, to such an extent that a popular movement against hospital delivery has gradually grown up. It began by putting pressure on doctors and midwives to improve the way that deliveries in hospital were carried out, starting with important but peripheral issues, such as not having pubic hair shaved for childbirth, a dangerous and dehumanizing practice, and then moved on to giving mothers a choice of the type of analgesia they would prefer and the freedom to choose the position in which to have the delivery. This has now built up to such a degree that it has persuaded the professionals to test the feasibility of the management of childbirth at home and is increasingly forcing them to allow it to occur in practice.

In the second half of this century home births in the USA, Canada and the UK passed from being a very small percentage to a negligible amount. Figure 5.6, taken from Torres and Reich [170], shows that the proportion of babies

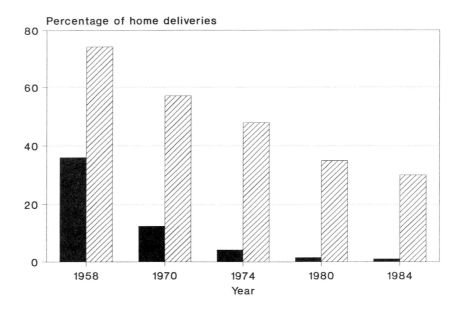

Figure 5.6 The UK (solid area) decreased its proportion of home deliveries very rapidly in the 1960s in contrast to The Netherlands (hatched area). Reproduced with permission from [170].

delivered at home fell rapidly during the 1960s and 1970s and remained low during the 1980s. In 1984, the maternity services advisory committee [171] encouraged all maternity care to be in hospital. Most births that did occur at home were unplanned.

The consensus for hospital care was broken within Europe by The Netherlands. In 1980, 35% of deliveries in The Netherlands took place at home. Although both the UK and The Netherlands increased their proportion of hospital births, the rates of change are very different. In addition, the perinatal mortality in The Netherlands was extremely low during this period (Figure 5.7).

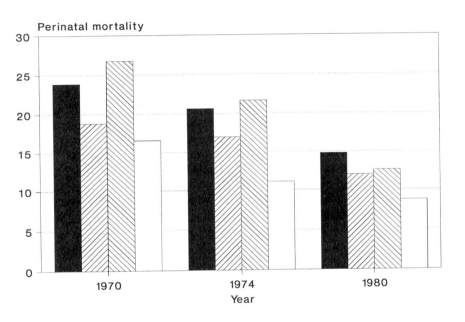

Figure 5.7 Perinatal mortality for England and Wales (■), The Netherlands (▨), West Germany (▧) and Sweden (□).

Comparisons between different countries are always fraught with traps for the unwary, but it is useful to look at the possible reasons for the difference in hospitalization in the UK and The Netherlands. This may give us a clue as to whether hospitals should continue to have the dominance that they hold over the maternity services against the clear preferences of a large proportion of their patients.

In The Netherlands, midwives are allowed to deliver babies in the home without medical supervision. They are also very involved in prenatal care and refer patients to physicians or hospitals if abnormalities arise. These midwives receive 3 years of professional training orientated towards midwifery whereas until very recently, British midwives had to be trained as general nurses for 3 years followed by 1 year of specialist obstetric training. An important reason for this difference appears to be that British midwives were displaced from practising prenatal care early in this century when medical practitioners, later consultants, developed outpatient maternity clinics and mobile units for emergencies outside hospital. The number of antenatal clinics increased from 120 in 1918 to total 1931 during World War II, and over three-quarters of pregnancies were supervised by physicians at that time.

With the development of the NHS in 1948, these policies had become accepted and were built into the new health service. It was expected that doctors would attend all births outside hospital and would be available for births in hospital. In The Netherlands, another group of people, the nursing aides, developed. These took care of healthy women and their children at home and assisted with housework. Their training lasted 15 months and included the study of hygiene, child care in the home and house care. Their training has been extended recently to include care of disabled people and the elderly.

It must be said that the obstetricians in The Netherlands favour hospital confinement and that in the last 20 years there has been a rapid rise in the number of obstetricians. Despite this rise in the number of consultants, the intervention rate in terms of caesarean sections and the use of anaesthetics in labour is still much lower in The Netherlands than in the UK.

One factor that almost certainly speeded up the move towards hospital care was the centralized planning apparatus of the health service, which was often stimulated into action by central committees, and a national policy which was regularly restated. The Ministry of Public Health in The Netherlands did not have a national policy on the place of birth. In addition, general practitioners in the UK are paid for the number of patients they have, not for what they do, and they therefore have no incentive to perform more deliveries. In The Netherlands, general practitioners are paid for what they do, encouraging them to carry out deliveries.

Private insurance in The Netherlands covers payment for prenatal care, delivery and postnatal care only if it is provided by the midwife and not the physician, as long as the midwife practices in the district and there are no medical indications for specialized care. If there is a midwife and there is no indication for specialized care any woman who wishes a physician to attend the delivery must pay for that attendance. This includes prenatal care.

In the UK, a number of national committees have made the connection between an increasing number of births in hospital and improvements in the perinatal mortality rate. However, there have always been detractors, who have suggested that the data have never supported such a wholesale move towards hospital care [172]. In the UK, it has been assumed that the safety of the mother and baby can only be assured if the birth occurs in hospital. Because of this it has also been assumed that women should not have a choice in where the birth should take place. There has been no scientific evidence to back up any of these beliefs. The dominance of the medical profession over the planning process when the health service was first set up ensured that consultants, who believed that hospital was the safest place for confinement, would increasingly have their views listened to.

It is now gradually becoming understood that institutional confinement can have adverse as well as positive consequences and that women should be able to choose. In the UK, the view has been that any risk, and all mothers and babies are at some risk, is completely unacceptable, no matter what the preferences of the parent might be.

It is interesting that no randomized controlled trials on maternity care given at home or in hospital were undertaken when these decisions were being made. In 1993, an attempt was made to do this, though the trial did not look at home deliveries *per se*, but built a unit in the hospital consisting of rooms similar to those found in a home to simulate home confinement [173].

One of the claimed benefits of hospital delivery has been the possibility of performing continuous monitoring of the baby before it is born. The benefits of such monitoring in low risk women have never been proved. The study simulating home care assigned over 2000 women to a midwife-led scheme and over 1000 to a consultant-led traditional scheme which had been used for some years. The women were randomly allocated to one scheme or the other. Three rooms near the delivery suite in Leicester Royal Infirmary were converted to appear like a normal household bedroom with carpeted floors, patterned wallpaper and matching curtains. The beds were of standard type and all the equipment, except that necessary for a normal delivery and resuscitation, was hidden behind curtains.

The suite was run entirely by the midwives who also ran the antenatal clinics. Some women who had had difficult previous births or had serious disease were excluded from the randomization as were those who were expecting twins. Just under half of all the women who came in for confinement during this period were entered into the study.

This study showed, using a large number of measures, that the women cared for in the homely environment were as safe as those treated in hospital. In addition, the women in the homely area of the hospital were considerably more satisfied with the care they had. This may have been owing to the novelty of the new unit, for staff and patients, but it is a finding that echoes throughout this book. Home or homelike care is sometimes a little safer than hospital care, sometimes a little cheaper, but is virtually always greatly preferred by patients.

CONSUMER POWER: ELDERLY PEOPLE IN THE USA

In Chapter 2 I mentioned the enormous pressure exerted by the American

Association of Retired Persons, which lobbied successfully to achieve medical cover for elderly people and a range of other benefits. The development of the organization was in response to the needs of elderly people for cheap insurance and other services, but the resulting group became very powerful politically.

There has not been an equivalent lobbying organization in the health care field in the UK. The nearest example of people 'voting with their feet' has been the development of private nursing homes in the UK in the 1980s. Elderly people who were poor found that entry to a private residential or nursing home was, in effect, free on demand. The number of private and residential homes increased over the decade by almost three times and private nursing homes by more than three times.

The advent of the Community Care Act in 1993 has altered the financial incentives, so that now elderly people who are poor can be supported in private institutions or at home. It has been estimated that just under two-thirds of the people who would be expected to go into residential homes, that is about a third of those who would be expected to go into nursing homes, are actually staying at home. These findings have not been confirmed by good research work as yet, but they show that given the opportunity to make choices which had previously been restricted for financial or other reasons, people are only to willing to take them up.

The examples I have cited have driven people into making particular choices because of the financial pressures on them. I believe that the advent of fund-holding general practitioners in particular and the development of the Patients' Charter within the health service may be the stimulus for the general public to realize that they can make choices, either by putting pressure on their general practitioner to request specific standards of care, or by refusing to use some hospital or community services that have a poor reputation.

INTERNATIONAL CONSUMER CHOICE

The most recent move by the UK government to take the preferences of patients seriously has been the Patients' Charter. Not surprisingly this has been derided by opposition political parties as a gimmick. Nevertheless, the possibilities posed by a central government commitment to consumer choice in the health service should not be treated lightly. In particular the charter promises to compensate patients for inefficient or unthinking care. This is discussed more fully in Chapter 10 on quality assurance. The main points of the charter that are likely to affect a patient's use of hospitals are:

● the right to change the family doctor
● the right to be referred to a consultant acceptable to the patient
● the right to be given a clear explanation of any treatment proposed and any alternatives before the patient decides whether to accept it.

It is suggested that, given that patients appear to prefer treatment in or near to their home, these rights will help to maintain the movement away from district general hospitals.

6	Effects of changes: prevention and assessment

PREVENTION IN THE COMMUNITY

Prevention of disease and maintenance of health are reasonably well developed in the UK, though they are still seen as being separate from the mainstream of medical services. The reasons for this are that health promotion and disease prevention are more to do with education than health. Health professionals should be, to some extent, teachers as well as being involved in therapy. However, most training schools for medical professionals are poorly organized for teaching their students how to sell health, how to teach professionals about advising patients, and how to help patients reduce their risks of getting ill. Health promotion and disease prevention are obviously important components of any plan for keeping people out of hospital. Hospital admission is, in some ways, a failure of the service.

There is therefore tension between the health and education services about who owns health education. It is certain that a great deal of health educational work is carried on outside the health service. In schools, a proportion of the courses in home economics, sport and biology are presented as health promotion. Thus, healthy eating and cooking permeates the home economics course, measures of heart and lung function are commonly used as measures of improvement in sports, especially athletics, and advice on drug abuse forms part of biology and science courses.

There are some dangers in using the avoidance of disease as a lever to persuade people to take part in these activities. First, the relationship between health and, for example, physical fitness is so little understood that individual cases of, for example, a well known sportsman or physically active politician dying young of heart disease can bring the whole theory into disrepute. Second, it seems a pity, especially in sport, to press an activity which some people find enjoyable and others loath onto the whole community for a very small long-term benefit to their heart and lungs.

The likelihood of reducing disease processes by changing people's lifestyle (usually meant to include what they eat, if they smoke, their sex lives and exercise) cannot be proved, even for groups of people. The most convincing evidence would be an experiment in which some individuals would be forced to take on an unhealthy lifestyle and others a healthy lifestyle. Recent suggestions that vegetarians live longer than meat eaters used a case control approach. For each vegetarian (case) in the study a relative or friend of that person was chosen who was a meat eater, 'the control' [174]. Even with the care taken in this study to try to take into account the known differences between the two groups there may well be a consistent difference in approach to life between meat eaters and non-meat eaters. The evidence remains strong but is still circumstantial.

However, if we alter the semantics and suggest that health is enhanced by changes in lifestyle there would be little disagreement. If health is related to a sense of 'complete physical, mental and social well-being' as defined by the WHO, or in a slightly less idealized form 'the ability to love and work' as defined by Freud, then an essential component of health is well-being. This is presumably enhanced by activities which are enjoyable. Indeed the statement becomes circular. A problem is that humans are prone to addiction, whether to sport, sex or muesli. Feeding the addiction may make them feel well but does not necessarily fit in with what most of us would regard as healthy.

It is to be hoped that evidence that generally contented people live longer [175] will be sufficient to allow the leisure industries to continue to act without recourse to detailed semi-scientific medical arguments about health to promote their ideas. It will not, of course, reduce the overall need for health services. Until any effective means of delaying the onset of disease is successful (a process which may take 20 years or more) the new preventive service will have to be financed at the same time as existing treatment services for disease.

Even accepting that the form of prevention is effective, short of eradicating the disease entirely the need for treatment for that disease will simply be delayed. In Chapter 2 I mentioned the possibility that as people live longer it seems likely that they will be less disabled at, say, 70 years of age. The question remains as to whether the balance between increasing numbers of very elderly people with their greater disability will be outweighed by a reduction in that disability as they get fitter at any one age. The result of that balance will decide whether more services are needed to care for them overall. This is not proven in either direction at present, but the small amount of evidence that does exist suggests relatively little change in the overall demands on the service.

The prevention of disease may enable people to live longer without disability, but it is still extremely unlikely to save money. The fact that we must all die sometime seems inevitably to mean that costs for the prevention of disease or the promotion of health must be added to those for treatment, not substituted for them. The only way around this would be if we restricted treatment for people past a certain age, or if the increased ageing of the population, due to prevention, was combined with an overall decrease in illness prior to death sufficient to outweigh the increased number of people.

It is unlikely therefore that the development of new health educational and promotional methods will, of themselves, be cost effective if, by this, we mean that they will reduce the number of people with disabilities and therefore their likely need for care. Health education and promotion are therefore not likely to alter the need for hospital care if the definition of who needs such care remains unchanged. Reductions in the number of places in hospital is more likely to be altered by changes in the policy for the admission of patients and reductions in their length of stay.

PEOPLE'S VIEWS ON THEIR OWN HEALTH

An important part of reducing the dependency of people on hospitals will be to reduce their psychological dependency on the model of illness and disease treatment from being something which is 'done somewhere else' to a feeling that they can contribute to their own care and treatment. This will require people to have a clearer view about illness and health.

There has been some research into people's views of their own health. This is extremely important when thinking about the future of all services, but especially those aimed at preventing illness. It is not the place of this book to go into detail about the sociological basis for health and disease. Suffice it to say that some people have a view of life in general, and health in particular, which suggests that they are able to control their own destiny, others do not [176].

An example of this is cited by Bandura who has suggested that there are variations in people's confidence to perform certain tasks in situations that the individual has not met before [177]. One could, for instance, ask someone who has never skied how well they would expect to be able to ski. Such a measure of self confidence is different from a real expectation of what will happen. Someone may have confidence in their ability to perform well at a job interview, but not expect that this would lead to employment because of other external factors, such as a belief that the job was already promised to someone else or that the interviewers might not appreciate their qualities. Such self confidence, or lack of it, is part of the personality of the person involved and does not seem to change much as people age, except in response to extremely traumatic events.

Men and women with and without such self confidence are different in their approach to health promotion and health education initiatives. Those who are highly self confident tend to behave in different ways about such things as smoking, exercise and weight control than those who are not. The former individuals seem to have a much stronger belief in their own ability to control their futures and may be more likely to follow advice from health professionals about improving or maintaining their health by, for instance, changing their diet [177a]. However, much of the work exploring the personality characteristics of people who are more or less likely to take advice has been restricted to young people and most of it has been performed in the USA. In the UK, the relationship between people's philosophy of life and their lifestyle has not often been studied.

One example of such work was carried out with more than 5000 people aged 17 and over in Cardiff [178]. They were asked about their lifestyle and their view of the degree of control that they felt they had over their lives. It was discovered that the responses these people made to the question 'Do you believe that health is almost all a matter of luck?' were a useful means of identifying groups of people who had different approaches to life and different reactions to health promotion messages.

Men and women were similar in their response to the question. Just under one in five felt that health is a matter of luck (the 'fatalists'), a further fifth were unable to decide. The rest, about two-thirds, felt that health was not a matter of luck and that one could influence it by one's own actions (the 'interventionists'). Figure 6.1 shows the distribution of the answers by the age and sex of the people answering the question.

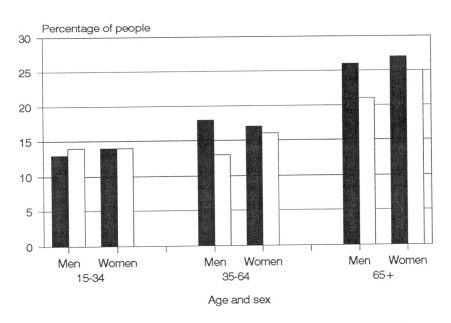

Figure 6.1 Older people are more likely to feel that health is a matter of luck. Some people felt health was a matter of luck (shaded); others were unsure (unshaded).

Older men and women showed an increasing tendency to agree with the statement, to be more fatalistic, and this trend was highly significant in each case. There was also a trend for older people to have more difficulty answering the question than younger people. When people were classified according to their occupation there was a close relationship between those with lower incomes and fatalism (Figure 6.2). This figure shows there is a trend for fatalism about health to be higher in the manual than non-manual occupations. If both occupational class and age are looked at together there is still a consistent trend for fatalism to increase with age. Thus the relationship between fatalism and age and fatalism and occupation appear to be independent of each other. About a third of unskilled workers over 65 years are fatalistic about their ability to control their own health.

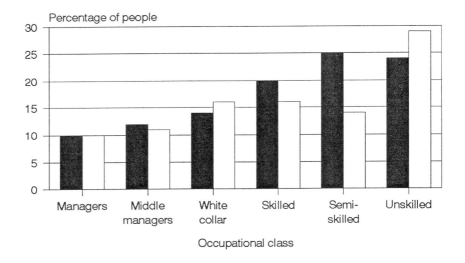

Figure 6.2 People with lower incomes are more likely to feel that health is a matter of luck. Those who agreed (shaded); those who were unsure (unshaded).

Figure 6.3 shows the relationship between fatalism and disability. There is a marked trend for disabled people to be more fatalistic. Older people also tend to be more disabled, so once again the figures were checked to make sure that the increased fatalism result was not confused by the older people being more disabled. Once again the two effects, in this case age and disability, were related to increasing fatalism independently of each other.

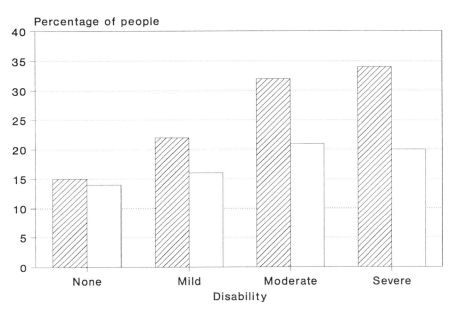

Figure 6.3 Disabled people are more likely to feel that health is a matter of luck. Those who felt that health was a matter of luck (shaded); those who were unsure (unshaded).

This approach to life appears to have a marked effect on the habits of people who are fatalistic, especially those habits thought to have an effect on health. Figure 6.4 shows that more of these people smoked. There was no effect on drinking, indeed a slightly lower percentage of those who were fatalistic drank alcohol. The group took less moderate exercise than others and were less likely to have altered their diet in the past year for the sake of their health.

Other information gathered during the survey showed that interventionists were more likely to have increased their intake of fish and fibre and reduced their intake of meat, sugar, fat and salt than others over the past year.

Overall, the study showed that those who feel that health is largely a matter of luck form a sizable minority of the population. They tend to be older, poorer and more disabled. Their view of life has a marked effect on some of their habits, notably smoking, exercise and diet. It is hard to know why the differences in fatalism for those with different degrees of poverty and disability exist. Previous work has shown people who are most knowledgeable about health in general are most likely to be taking a conventionally defined healthy diet [179].

For elderly and disabled people such a 'healthy diet' has not really been clearly defined. It may be, for instance, that reducing fat and increasing fibre

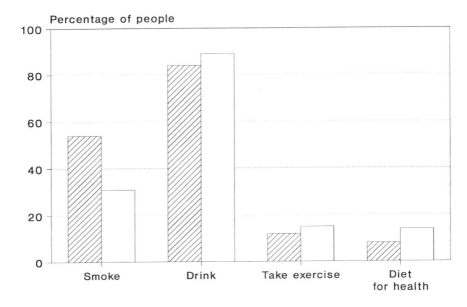

Figure 6.4 Lifestyle is affected by attitude to health. Fatalists (shaded); interventionists (unshaded).

intake may have a deleterious effect on vitamin D intake. It is certainly likely that a lack of guidelines, such as those recently published by the King's Fund [180], has hampered workers in the field and led to disillusion for elderly and disabled people. These men and women feel disfranchised from society in general; this includes messages for health promotion, which often portray the aim of their work as being to maintain young, fit, beautiful and beautifully dressed people in their enviable state. It is little wonder that such messages are rejected by poor, disabled and elderly citizens.

In the USA, advice for elderly people has been available for some time, from the Surgeon General. This has been in the form of a programme specifically aimed at older individuals and includes reduction of smoking, provision of exercise opportunities, nutrition guidance and assistance [181]. Good evidence on the effectiveness of the last two does not really exist, but at least there is an agreed policy in the USA which can be argued about.

People working for the health and social services can easily discourage older and poorer people with unfriendly attitudes [182]. It may be these attitudes that cause elderly people, the poor and the disabled to feel that they have little control over their own health. It is known, for instance, that older people are often ignorant of the health-related services available to them [124], which must result in their having less confidence in those services than younger people.

Perhaps the most important factor is to do with expectations. For example, young people feel old age will be the worst period of their life [183]. This expectation is established early on [184] and is, in general, shared by old people about their peers [185]. Small wonder then that older people tend to regard the maintenance of their health with fatalism.

The message for health promoters is clear. There needs to be a strategy developed for health promotion in poor, disabled and older people and this needs to be as clearly and enthusiastically developed as that for the mainstream. It seems particularly obtuse that the poorest, oldest and most disabled people, known to be most at risk from disease and further disability, are not searched out. It would seem sensible to customize the work done by health promotion so that it reaches these groups in particular.

PREJUDICES TO BE OVERCOME

Taking control of one's own health, which is likely to be a central part of moving from hospital to home-based services, will, at first, be uncomfortable. The process of health promotion and disease prevention includes the danger of allowing the health industry (represented at its most powerful by general hospitals) to invade the whole of life. Medicine can so easily meddle in sport, eating or sex. On the other hand, some people are excluded from useful and important information and assistance because of a paternalistic attitude of society about how much control over their own lives some groups should be allowed. The following examples, which illustrate the point, relate to children and elderly people.

Health education in children; too much knowledge?

Health promotion and education often give what appear to be political messages. This is because they usually aim to cover populations, rather than individuals, and give messages which often stray away from people with overt illness into the fields of family life and individual versus group responsibilities. These can often cause clashes in society. The main areas of contention centre around issues of poverty or, in the UK, sex, and its effect on health.

The AIDS epidemic, a fatal disease, the incidence of which can be alleviated by health education, has caused direct clashes between health educators and politicians. The educators are aware of the terrifying consequences of not stopping the epidemic, and therefore give advice on sexual matters in language that is unmistakable. The politicians, responding to their own and their shocked constituents' sensibilities, appear to believe that talking about sex, especially to children, is the main factor which leads them to experiment sexually. As a result, health educators regularly find their latest advice confiscated as if it were pornography while the government funds its own awareness campaigns.

Elderly people and smoking: their only pleasure?

Publications on helping elderly people to stop smoking tend to be bland in the extreme, with comments on smoking being one of the 'few remaining pleasures' for elderly people [186]. A number of textbooks on health promotion [187] and a WHO Advisory Group on health promotion in elderly people [188] have omitted the subject entirely. However, Americans are more convinced of the importance of such an approach [189], though comments on its benefits are confined to potential increases in longevity.

Despite considerable opposition, including difficulties with getting funding, I eventually persuaded a charitable trust to assist me with a study on the subject [190]. Just over 2500 people aged 60 and over, in a large general practice, were contacted and cigarette smokers were identified. The people who were cigarette smokers were randomly allocated to two groups. Each member of one group was invited to go and see his or her general practitioner who asked if he or she would like to stop smoking and explained the importance of giving up, especially the potential benefits of feeling better. Each person was then given the opportunity to discuss the possible problems associated with stopping smoking with a nurse who had had experience of smoking clinics for all age groups.

The nurse undertook a general health promotion approach offering advice on lifestyle in general, but concentrating on assistance with giving up smoking. This was carried out at a weekly clinic which went on for 6 months. Interestingly, the clinic became popular with other age groups who wanted to give up smoking and a number of younger people were referred to it by the general practitioners.

Half of the cigarette smokers were offered this special clinic, the other half were not. Figure 6.5 shows the proportion of people who were smoking 6 months after the clinics had finished. People in both groups had stopped smoking to some extent, but those who were offered the clinic had reduced their smoking more than the ones who were not. All of those who claimed to have stopped were checked by having their breath tested using a carbon monoxide monitor. For all age groups, a higher proportion of the clinic group stopped smoking when compared with the control group. The proportion stopping in both groups fell with increasing age from about a fifth of those aged 60–64 to less than a tenth of those aged 75 and over. More important than giving up smoking was the finding that there was a significant reduction in the amount of breathlessness suffered by the group who had been offered the facilities of the clinic compared with those who had not. Stopping smoking had a rapid effect on reducing their symptoms.

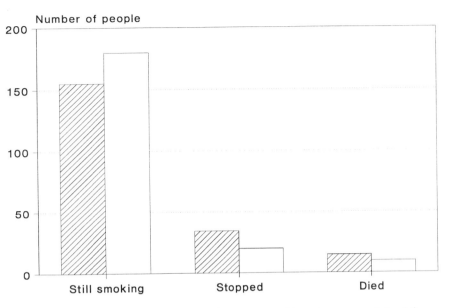

Figure 6.5 Elderly people were more likely to stop smoking when a nurse helped them to do so (shaded) than an identical group that did not have such help (unshaded).

In order to find out whether those who stopped smoking had suffered symptoms due to the process of stopping itself another comparison was made between those who stopped and those who did not. Symptoms caused by stopping smoking have been described as trembling, nausea and irritability. It was suspected that stopping smoking might have had such adverse effects on some people. In fact people who continued to smoke showed a worsening of these symptoms compared with those who stopped. Despite these generally positive findings there was considerable reluctance on the part of some of the general practitioners in the study to refer their patients for help in stopping smoking. This was particularly noticeable for patients who were disabled. They were considered to have enough problems without attempting to give up smoking as well.

Approaches to health education and promotion are firmly rooted in community care, but many of the benefits of the approach can be dissipated by its social features. These problems highlight the relatively high profile that health matters have when they are delivered to the community, whether in school or in people's homes. As a result, the care given in the community needs to be acceptable, not simply to the people involved, but often to the general population. Health promotion messages or assistance to stop smoking in hospital will hardly be noticed. Once care is given in the community it becomes the property of the whole population.

ASSESSMENT IN THE COMMUNITY

Hospitals have the advantage of a wide range of different professionals providing their services under the same roof. The benefit of this for treating patients is that the services which patients need do not have to be planned far in advance. A patient in hospital can have any of these services provided at the bedside or in the relevant department, simply by calling that department. Departments are often unaware of what their workload is going to be and therefore have got into the habit of having staff available in case of an increase in demand. The result of this is that facilities in hospital have less pressure on them to plan ahead than do community based services. If there are insufficient or badly managed services this leads to internal waiting lists. If there are too many services they tend to be more costly than they need to be, to allow for the flexibility of always having the service available.

A number of studies, notably those drawn together by a recent Audit Commission report [191], have shown that many hospitals suffer from this lack of forward planning. It is well illustrated by data about when to discharge a patient from hospital. It has been suggested that good initial assessment and planned management of patients will help to overcome this inefficiency. My own contention is that planning and management of patients' conditions in other settings, whether at home, in a general practitioner's surgery or a small specialist unit, will allow better assessment and management of the care of that patient than exists at present. Also, because of the nature of the service, it will have to be well planned and therefore have smaller waiting lists.

Assessment and care management by the family

Some work has suggested that the more education and information care givers get about looking after their relatives, the less strain and the more well-being that relative will feel [192]. Research in the USA has shown how family members can be directly involved in the care of disabled people in a more constructive way than simply acting as an adjunct of, or alternative to, services. Their aim is to link closely the paid service suppliers with families so that they can help each other. Both the family and the services have the same plan, though they may operate on different principles. That plan is to assist a dependent person. Care management acts as a way of making links between families and social services or health workers.

Trials have been conducted to test how well this can work [193]. The first study was set up to discover how useful it would be to train family members to do the care management for their relative. Training the family to take more control reduced their need to use the paid for services [194]. The study concentrated on a group of semi-dependent elderly people in a well off suburb of Boston. Another study was set up, by the same group, to look at whether such training for relatives would work for more dependent people. It also looked at the effect of the training on the relationship between different relatives and between the relatives and the patient.

The second study looked at two groups, the family members of people who were on renal dialysis and another group who were looking after patients with dementia. Half of the relatives were given assistance, the others acted as controls to test how well the approach worked. There were discussions and direct hands on training about the emotional and practical problems of caring for a relative and the special needs of the family care givers. The purpose was to allow the family members to work better with and understand the paid for services and what they were trying to do and to understand more fully the disease process afflicting their relative including its complications and likely outcome.

The families who were given training were able to organize themselves to assist social services, nurses and those providing transportation for the patient better than those who were not trained. When patients were admitted to hospital, discharge was earlier than for the group with the untrained relatives. There appeared to be little difference between the group given training and those who were not when their feelings about caring for their dependent relative were examined, but the relationships within the family were better for those who had the intervention.

HOW MANY PEOPLE NEED TO BE IN HOSPITAL?

The most important part of assessment for patients prior to going into hospital is the decision about whether such an admission is really needed. Inpatient care is extremely expensive, so this decision is also critical for the costs of services. Research groups have shown that a high proportion of the people in hospital should not have been admitted and that many stay longer than is necessary.

One of the most dramatic of these studies [195] showed that almost two-thirds of patients in 847 general medical and surgical beds did not need to be in the acute hospital bed they occupied.

This study is not unique, work in the USA [196] and in the UK [197, 198] has shown similar results, but the Anderson et al. study [195] is important to the subject of this book, so it is worth looking at in a little more detail. The authors looked at nearly 850 admissions to the John Radcliffe Hospital in Oxford over a 3 week period. They developed and used a questionnaire aimed at measuring whether the patients in the hospital were being kept there appropriately. The questionnaire was similar to the Boston appropriateness evaluation protocol

[199] which measured unnecessary days of hospital care. The group of patients studied excluded those in the obstetric, gynaecological and children's departments.

The patient was considered to have a positive reason to be in hospital if any of the following criteria were met:

- a life threatening condition needing treatment or observation
- invasive therapeutic or investigation that day
- postoperative day for above
- monitoring by doctor
- ventilated
- intravenous therapy
- major wound care
- monitoring vital signs
- preoperative evaluation for invasive procedure.

Using this questionnaire it was found that only four out of 10 patients should have been using the bed on the day that they were questioned: only four of every 10 patients had a positive reason for being in hospital.

When these data were looked at in more detail it was found that about half of the surgical beds were filled for positive reasons, in contrast to just over a third of the medical beds, and less than a quarter of the geriatric beds. The proportion of beds filled for positive reasons was related to the patients' age. Half of the patients under 65 had positive reasons for filling a bed compared with only a fifth of those 85 and over. The proportion of beds positively filled also decreased from three-quarters on the first day (suggesting that a quarter were wrongly admitted) to one-fifth on the eighth day after admission.

The proportion of people occupying a bed for positive reasons on any one day was closely related to the days consultants took their ward rounds. On the day leading up to a consultant round the proportion was very low (a third). This increased on the day after the ward round to just under two-thirds. This suggests that a large number of patients were simply waiting for the consultant to give them permission to leave.

Figure 6.6 shows details of the patients who were there and why. The commonest positive reason for being in hospital was the need for specialist skills. The commonest reason for not being sent home, when a patient could have been, was the need for nursing care. With the developments mentioned already in this book it can be seen that virtually all of the categories could be managed outside hospital with the possible exception of activities for life threatening disease. Fewer than one in 20 of the people assessed fall into this category. The patients undergoing invasive procedures could, at present, mostly be seen as day patients. If this proved to be impossible for, say, half of them, the total number needing hospital stay at present, using available techniques, would still be fewer than one in 10. Given the pressures I have outlined they are very likely to be treated at home in future.

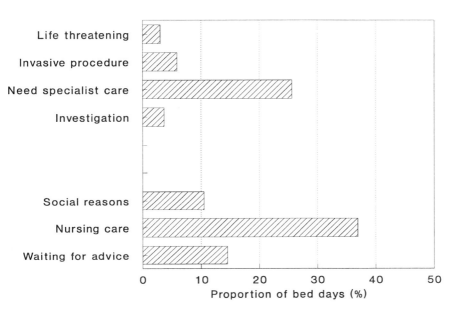

Figure 6.6 Proportion of bed days spent in hospital for various reasons. Reproduced with permission from [195].

This suggests that with better community services, including the availability of specialist help, nine out of 10 patients could, given the present state of knowledge, be managed without hospital care.

It has been shown that it is reasonably easy to reach agreement on suitable lengths of stay for different groups of patients [200] and to reduce inappropriate bed usage [201] if good admission criteria and discharge planning are in place. The Anderson *et al.* study in Oxford [195] showed that there was little evidence of either of these in practice in a renowned teaching hospital. Thus, without any changes in technique or improvements in technology, the length of stay in hospital could be dramatically reduced by improving planning.

DEVELOPING ASSESSMENT OF NEEDS IN THE COMMUNITY

Health care professionals assess their patients when they first see them. This assessment is critical and should lead to a discussion between the professional and the patient about what is likely to be wrong, the chances of its being helped and preferably a range of options from which the patient may choose, with the pros and cons of each spelled out. This is the care management process mentioned earlier in this chapter. If the patient is, or is likely to become, dependent this discussion needs to include other members of the family and other professional groups.

At present, the majority of these assessments are made by general practitioners in the patient's home. General practitioners are trained to look for a particular range of problems, particularly those which are biomedical. They are not very skilled at spotting problems which fall outside this range. Evidence for this was gathered in a survey of people at home aged 70 and over [201a]. The general practice in question has an excellent reputation in the area, particularly in its work with older people. Over 600 people aged 70 and over, living at home, were studied by a nurse employed for the purpose. The problems the nurse detected, using a comprehensive assessment of the elderly people, are shown in Figure 6.7. It can be seen that a wide range of problems were discovered, most of them physical in nature, but with mental, social, environmental and carer problems all making an important contribution.

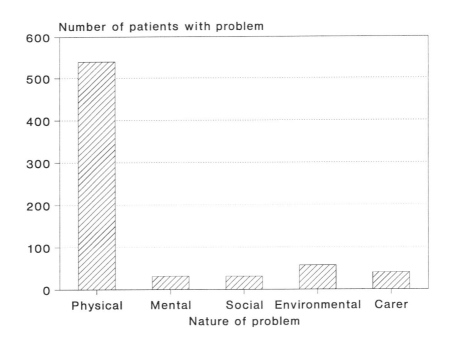

Figure 6.7 Problems suffered by people aged 70 years and over detected by a nurse visiting their home.

The next stage was to look at whether or not these problems had been noted previously by the general practitioner. This was assessed in two ways, by looking at the practice notes and also by questioning the general practitioners and other practice staff directly about individual patients known to have these problems. Figure 6.8 shows that the general practitioners were aware of seven out of 10 of the physical problems detected by the health visitor, two-thirds of the mental afflictions, but far fewer social and environmental problems and carer difficulties.

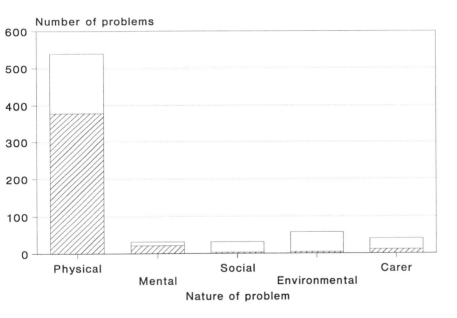

Figure 6.8 Problems previously detected by the general practitioner (shaded) and those not detected (unshaded).

The most important specific problems, classified as physical and most commonly missed by the general practitioners, were difficulties caused by feet. These are especially important in old people as such problems can cause immobility. The research nurse detected 34 people with active problems with their feet but the general practitioners were aware of only four. Two other important spheres where the general practitioners missed active physical problems were eyesight where just 15 out of 36 of those with difficulties had been detected and hearing deficits where only 12 out of 29 had been detected. Other important physical problems undetected by general practitioners when compared with the research nurse were frequent falls and severe urinary symptoms; the latter represented by 10 females with incontinence of whom only five had been recognized.

These findings could have been an artefact due to incomplete note taking and the poor memories of the general practitioners when asked if they already knew about a problem. However, this seems unlikely, as they had high rates of knowledge about specific medical conditions. As an example, 44 out of 46 people with active heart disease were known to the general practitioners, using the same method of checking.

Two-thirds of mental problems were previously known to the general practitioners. There was no particular pattern of those best detected. However, all four cases of severe depression had been noticed by the general practitioners. For those with social problems only a tenth had previously been detected by the general practitioner. Social difficulties were usually caused by family rejection, noisy neighbours or isolation. There was no particular pattern about the types that were not noticed by the general practitioners; most were not noticed.

Problems classified as environmental were, in a similar way, very poorly detected. Poor housing conditions, difficulty with getting to an inaccessible toilet and not being able to bath because the bathroom was upstairs and the patient relatively immobile were rarely noticed. One particular problem was the difficulty some elderly people had in getting to their doctor; not surprisingly perhaps, this was completely undetected.

A third of the carers who had problems were identified by the general practitioners as being in trouble. The commonest specific problem found by the nurse was a main carer who was old and disabled and therefore unable to give adequate care to the patient. The general practitioner noticed 10 cases out of 29 where this was the main problem facing the family.

It was possible that the problems uncovered by the nurse, but not detected by the general practitioner, were relatively trivial and therefore not worthy of note; the nurse may have been making a fuss about nothing. In order to check this, problems were classified into those that were thought to be mild, moderate or severe. Figure 6.9 shows the results for those classified as severe only.

Four out of 10 of the physical problems were previously known to the general practitioner. This is a considerably smaller proportion than the seven out of 10 problems of all severity known by them. It appears that the general practitioners were less aware of the severe problems affecting their elderly patients, including those based on physical problems.

This suggests that the nurse was not uncovering a series of unknown trivial problems, but, because of her more intensive method of working, was detecting many of the complex socio-medical problems so important to the care of patients, especially those with chronic disease. It is possible that these problems were not discovered by the general practitioners because of the narrow biomedical nature of their training.

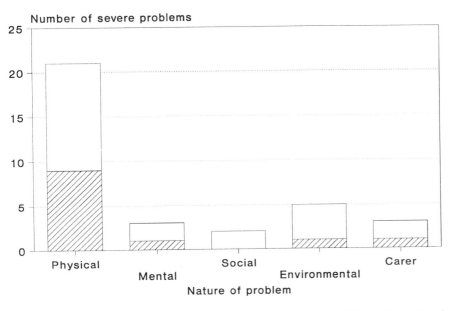

Figure 6.9 Severe problems previously detected by the general practitioner (shaded) and those not detected (unshaded).

LIMITATIONS OF THE MARKET APPROACH FOR ASSESSMENT

The community care part of the NHS and Community Care Act 1990 aimed to make it possible to care for mentally ill, learning disabled, and physically disabled people, both young and old, flexibly and with consciousness of the resources available. In order to accomplish this, much reliance has been put on an effective method of assessing and managing the care of patients.

The phrase 'assessment and care management' is a technical way of deciding what a patient needs and delivering it, in agreement with the patient, his or her family and the professionals who are likely to be involved in the care. The centre point of this system is that the service provider, most commonly a nurse or social worker, makes an assessment of what the patient or client needs. This provider has to have the necessary authority to call on a wide range of services and, more importantly, a wide range of providers of those services from health, social services, housing and the private or voluntary agencies [202].

This could include, for example, asking a neighbour to come in each morning to make up a fire, having a postman regularly check that an isolated disabled person is well, providing cooking classes to an elderly man who has never learned to look after himself, finding volunteers to read to a blind person, or obtaining nursing care for treating a chest infection in a patient who is severely disabled.

Such an approach comprises five stages: screening, assessing, planning, managing and monitoring. Screening is an essential part of the process because many people who require assistance need basic and uncomplicated care. The development of the internal market within the health and social services, if it gives more power to consumers, could make such work unnecessary. Patients could, if given the chance, simply choose the services they wanted from a list of competing providers.

Such an approach for providing health care was not felt to work well for disabled people. Many disabled people, even if they could afford it, may have difficulty in identifying and getting in touch with the right services. For this reason it was felt to be important to set up good assessment services for all groups of dependent people: the mentally ill, people with learning disability and people who are physically disabled, of all ages. This would allow patients to discuss the available options with a professional who understood the system, usually known as a 'key worker'. However, the key worker will, to some extent, act as a barrier to patients obtaining services. This must be recognised, for there has been a tendency for assessment to become ceremonial in its complexity and an end in itself.

The forgotten first step: screening and case finding

Screening is an essential part of any plan so that the people who are providing services can decide whether the caller has a problem that can be improved by their services [203]. Screening can often be completed by a telephone call and is set up to decide whether the caller is eligible for the service and whether a further assessment will better define what exactly the caller needs. A high proportion of patients can be sorted out at the screening stage with advice or the provision of a simple one-to-one service.

The screening system set up in the UK varies from area to area but usually measures 'functional and cognitive abilities' of patients, that is what they can do and what they can understand. It aims to measure, reasonably objectively, the severity of the patient's problem. In the UK, this is not simply for deciding which type of service should be provided. If the patient is defined by the screening process as requiring health care, that care will be given free of charge, if social care is required the patient will have to pay for it, unless he or she is poor.

I have mentioned that many problems can be solved at the screening stage without further assessment. However, a number of service providers in the UK fail to use a screening procedure at all during their initial contact. This is foolish and wasteful. It is theorized that patients may not be aware of what is available or their own degree of need. If this is true the right approach is to make available to the public the essential information that all clients or patients require before they even approach services, but the patients' lack of awareness is not a good enough excuse for not using a screening procedure.

Assessment

Once screening has been completed an assessment is made which is used as the basis for planning. This usually consists of a systematic protocol with a number of scales. A great number of these have been developed in different places. It appears that in the UK, due to the requirement for the Community Care Act to be implemented by local agreements between the local health authorities and social services departments almost every district has developed a different system. The assessments are usually set up to allow a number of different disciplines to use one centralized method with regard to the questions and subject matter included. The assessment may be completed by more than one person but because of the cost that this entails a single individual is usually chosen to give the assessment. A variety of measures of cognitive ability and sometimes emotional state may be used.

It is important to realize that this assessment may give a view of the severity of the problems which the client or patient may have. However, it does not take the place of, for example, a personalized medical assessment. For deciding on a plan of action in complex cases the assessment often simply forms the core of the information necessary, rather than being sufficient on its own.

Planning care

This involves translating the problems and needs identified in the assessment into assistance or training for the patient or client. The process is largely a negotiation between the client's preferences, interests and abilities and the view of the professionals about the problem, how it can be tackled and what is likely to be achieved as a result of that. Part of the planning process is the cost of the services to be provided and who should pay for them, the client, the person providing the service or someone else. At this stage patients should be given a choice of options.

There are problems. Some studies have shown that clients who had previously agreed to what was put on their plan said that they had not really understood the options and once informed fully of the many services that they might choose from said that they would have chosen differently [204]. The planning process should also try to take into account the interests and wishes of the family. It has been suggested in some places that family members themselves can act as case managers for their relatives arranging services and monitoring their quality [205]. Other people have suggested that dependent people with any degree of mental competence could, given good information about the pros and cons of different services and the amount of money available, organize, manage and monitor their own care.

In order to avoid the difficulties of budgeting at this stage it has been suggested that elderly people who are able to plan their own care might be given vouchers which would cover a range of services and which they could supplement out of their own pocket. For the majority of disabled and/or elderly people, a reasonable retirement pension would allow them to make their own decisions about what services they wanted; as fewer of them would then need income support they could simply buy in their own assistance.

It might be thought that forecasting the cost of care plans for a group of clients would be difficult when the care manager is not aware of the needs of all his or her clients. However, with training, reliable cost projections do seem to be possible. In other words care managers are able to ration what they provide and make reasonable estimates of what will be needed in the future. This high-lights a problem of care managers: on the one hand, they act as an information source for the person needing care and a protagonist on their behalf; on the other, they have a duty to ration the money available to individuals in order to allow the rest of their group of clients to receive the assistance they need.

It might be said that all professionals who are not in an open market for their services (where patients pay them directly) have this dichotomy in mind, if only in relation to their own time. The more they give one patient the less they have for others. This can be seen at its most obvious in a busy outpatient department. The more time a consultant spends with one patient, the longer the rest have to wait. This has been mentioned as a specific problem for community care. Often the decisions about the use of resources are taken by relatively junior members of staff without direct supervision. This is a new problem for them. Senior consultants and social workers in the UK are used to having to ration them-selves and the services they can call on and feel this paradox less acutely.

Monitoring the care

Care managers need to keep closely in touch with their patients to assure them-selves that promised services do in fact arrive and are altering the situation for the better. Part of the monitoring process should take the form of an assessment at intervals. This has been particularly lacking in the UK where, for instance, in residential homes for elderly people and geriatric long term care units there is a tendency for patients to stay for life once admitted.

DOES IT ALL WORK?

There have been a number of studies estimating the cost effectiveness of assess-ment and care, often called care management. There is a general consensus that the system can be extremely expensive, particularly if a detailed assessment is carried out in the majority of cases. One such enquiry in the USA, the triage experiment [206] carried out in 1981, had available a wide range of medical, transportation and visiting services. It was also concerned with deciding whether patients required outpatient, nursing home or hospital care.

In general, the programme evaluators felt that triage was a more expensive way of allocating care than allocating community care in the normal way. Previously each professional assessed what the patient or client needed and provided for those needs directly with no attempt to develop multidisciplinary teams beyond the normal relationships and friendships between different professionals in the same area. There was no advantage for the clients in terms of well-being in one group or the other.

Another programme, in Georgia, compared the usual community care treatment programmes with a care management system. In this study, it was found that the original system had fewer deaths and used fewer nursing home places. Another project, in San Francisco in 1985 [207], had no effect on the function of the patients, their continence or their ability to perform activities of daily living, though they were slightly better at coping at home.

Despite this long history of research using good trials in the USA, there have been no randomized controlled trials of care management in the UK. The best known study, which was a case control study and therefore more open to bias, was performed in Kent [202] at about the same time as the triage work. It suggested that care management was more cost effective than the traditional approach, but strongly stressed the need for a careful screening process before committing a lot of money to assessment.

DISTANCE MONITORING

Health workers in the field can be supported by the use of communications technology. This has been called 'telemedicine'. It is defined as the practice of health care delivery using an interactive audiovisual communication system without the usual physical contact between health worker and patient [208]. Several groups in the USA and Canada tried out such systems during the 1950s and 1960s. These approaches were speeded up during the late 1960s by the development of the National Aeronautics and Space Administration (NASA) programmes which created the need to transmit medical data from the crew of spacecraft to earth.

Similar communication techniques were used in the Arizona desert for Papago Indians to send information back from their remote communities to primary health care facilities. Other techniques which have used satellites to transmit information include X-rays and other images. These have been tried in Alaska, north-west Ontario in Canada, and in remote parts of Japan. Telemedicine has therefore, so far, been confined to remote areas with long distances between the patient and the health worker. A more recent approach has been described by Watson [209]. This was set up using a network which involved the use of a satellite link in Australia. To start with, small inpatient units used the system to contact their base regional hospitals and to get second opinions as well as to question patients.

The equipment also allowed for faxing and for sending scanning images of patients, X-ray films and ultrasound images to other areas. In future it is likely that a television link will be possible, reasonably cheaply, using basic telephone equipment to communicate between rural general practitioners' surgeries or inpatient units and central specialists. This could transmit advice on laboratory results, diagnosis or treatment. Such systems can be used for setting up conferences to decide on the best approach for particularly difficult cases or to work out guidelines for the treatment of different problems.

Monitoring patients in their normal environment

A number of monitors that collect information directly from the patient and store or send that information to a central point by radio already exist and are likely to increase in popularity. Monitoring of heart rhythm has been carried out in this way for some years [210]. They are often able to elicit subtle changes in a patient's physiology which routine testing in hospital is unable to do. A number of daily activities, for example, have been discovered to be more stressful than was thought using hospital tests. These include driving to work and speaking with one's lawyer or bank manager. In the early stages many such assessments will be carried out at outpatient or day units attached to hospitals, but as techniques improve attendance at such facilities will not be needed.

More and more such work is being carried out either in primary care or in community based units. The latter are variously derived. They may be small general practitioner hospitals, sometimes known as community, neighbourhood or locality hospitals. They may be based on social services team headquarters, but containing a number of health professionals, especially nurses and therapists. Some are based in day hospitals or day centres, which are free-standing in the community. Whatever their origins these centres are gradually taking on more and more of the work of hospitals or acting as bases for people working in patients' homes.

7

Effects of changes: cure

CURATIVE APPROACHES IN COMMUNITY CARE

The sort of problems inherent in the move from hospital to home care are well described in the Tomlinson report [211] on the future of health care in inner London and the government's and the general public's response to that report [212]. The report is widely known for its attempt to sort out the problems of London's hospitals. The description of the present primary care system, which is the more central part of the report, suggests that London does not compare well with other English inner cities for its general practitioner services.

Tomlinson proposed 'development zones' for improving the primary and community care services in London. For this, the report drew evidence from a number of pilot projects and experiments about improving primary care services. Many of them have important messages about moving from hospital to home care in other parts of the UK. The relationship between primary, secondary, institutional and community services was one example. Figure 7.1 shows one way of describing the relationship between them on two axes, one from primary care to secondary care, the other from community to institutional care.

Primary care, meaning services that patients can get access to directly, varies in the degree to which it is entirely or partially based in institutions or the community. The quadrant which is rapidly developing new approaches to the treatment of patients is secondary care in the community. New services tend to be less compartmentalized than older ones. The spectrum between purely community services and purely institutional on the one hand and purely primary or purely secondary on the other is increasingly becoming blurred.

Tomlinson, in his report, suggested a checklist for improving primary and community services. This included bringing existing services up to scratch and looking at services which are particularly important in one locality because of the nature of the local population (for example, if the local area contains many homeless people or people from ethnic minorities) and expanding these improvements to all community and primary care services. The programme to put right existing flaws in the service included some straightforward

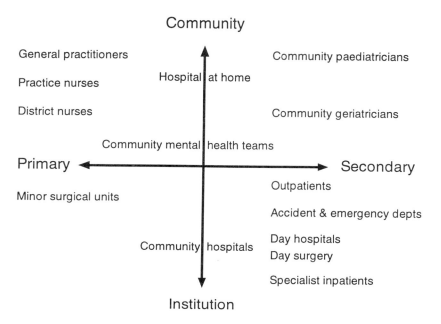

Figure 7.1 Relationship between health services.

approaches, such as looking at methods of attracting good general practitioners to the area and assisting others to take early retirement. It also included improving the physical layout and structure of premises and strengthening the links between primary and secondary services, both in the community and in hospital.

An important general aspect of community care was touched on with a suggestion for providing a set of core services in each area but with new ideas being tried out in different zones, depending on the nature of the specific problems in that zone. By their nature, local services are small scale and can therefore take risks with the type of service that each provides. They are able to aim at specific groups who might normally receive little attention, such as people from ethnic minorities, homeless people, mobile families and homosexuals. Tomlinson suggests, and the logic seems reasonable, that institutions are much less helpful to people in inner cities than in other places. However, the same argument would apply to any community which had unusual problems. Indeed it may be said that all small communities have special characteristics and that primary and community services should be tailored to those particular peculiarities.

A number of possible solutions to these problems have been suggested in the past, such as sick bays for homeless and indigent people, the use of salaried general practitioners where the population is constantly changing, specialist community nurses for families in bed and breakfast accommodation, interpretation and advocacy services for people in ethnic minorities, and outreach teams for people who are abusing drugs, or living on the streets or in hostels. Other suggestions have included ambulatory care centres where a range of walk in services are available including specialist clinics, diagnostic facilities and minor surgery.

This approach is simply a way of reorganizing primary and community care so that it is more customized to the particular needs of the local community. It is not a radical development of what already exists. It is simply an acknowledgement that large hospitals are not particularly well suited to providing flexible types of care for groups of people who have uncommon medical needs.

The next step Tomlinson suggested was to expand the model of primary and community care for homeless people so that much of the work presently done by hostels, with little or no contact with other organizations, is made part of the other health and social services. This requires close collaboration between general practitioners and community or hospital based consultants for the diagnosis and treatment of common conditions. Community nurses, in particular, will have to work in a number innovative ways, some of which they may find restrictive as they will be working, unusually, directly with consultants.

Tomlinson suggested the development of hospital at home and other high intensity home care schemes, developments in paediatric home care, mental health and learning disabilities teams, the use of general practitioner beds in community hospitals, and beds in small units run by nurses or nurse practitioners. He went on to suggest that much of the terminal care at present based in hospices and hospitals could be performed in the community. He suggested, in line with changes in care of mental illness, learning disability and paediatric patients, that much hospital outpatient work could be done in collaboration with or on the premises of general practitioners and community nurses.

In setting up the Tomlinson model of development zones it has been suggested that health authorities will have to decide, with general practitioners, the services that are needed to ensure that they are in place. This will need to be done at a local level. It is interesting that many of the changes suggested have been highlighted by the financial pressures on London's hospitals.

Possibly the most fascinating aspect of the Tomlinson report was the extent to which all of these important facets of the work were completely ignored by the media. Newspaper and television coverage of the proposals focused on which hospitals were likely to close as a result of the changes. Whether the resulting campaigns for saving different hospitals were led by people with vested interests in the hospitals, were a reflection of the natural conservatism of Londoners, or a spontaneous demonstration of the affection that local people felt for a loved and trusted institution is difficult to tell. It may be that people were concerned about the possibility of privatization by the 'back door' or that there was a feeling of uncertainty about what would replace the hospitals. It did demonstrate an important difficulty with bringing about any changes which require a move from hospital to community care.

A similar move towards the planning and delivery of services in small populations, known variously as neighbourhoods or localities, is developing in many health authorities and commissions who are purchasing services in the UK. One reason for this is to simplify the coordination of planning between the health authority commissioners and the local general practitioners, whether fundholders or not. This development of small area planning is therefore resulting from two completely different pressures: the need to coordinate general practitioners and the need to develop alternative services to reduce the dependence on acute hospital care.

The common factor is the need to reduce our dependence on hospitals in the health service. An important benefit of not having the hospital as a central point is that one is not bound to make planning areas as big as the catchment area of the hospital. The population sizes for large hospitals need to be at least a quarter of a million people to provide a good range of services. Without the constraints of needing to serve a hospital, planning services can be reduced to population sizes which better reflect communities with common problems. The planning area can therefore reflect the problems of the community, not the pressure to find enough patients to fill beds.

Another factor which these changes have in common is a suggestion that more of the work should be done at the primary care level, by general practitioners and their primary health care team. Figure 7.1 suggests that specialists in a number of disciplines (certainly mental illness, learning disability, the care of elderly people and the care of children) will be widespread through the community. These will form the community based secondary services. Other specialists (surgeons and general physicians) will increasingly hold their outpatient departments in community facilities. These will usually be in general practice premises, allowing useful contacts between the specialists and the general practitioners. Development of 'hospital at home' services and ambulatory day surgical units for a wide range of illnesses and the preoperative work of routine surgical cases will mean that the centrally situated hospitals will concentrate on intensive care, the management of major injuries and acute surgical emergencies. Training, except for these specific specialties, will be carried out in the community.

THE 'HOSPITAL AT HOME' SCHEMES

There are a number of ways of setting up acute hospital care at home. If good community services already exist, hospitals at home may be an offshoot of those services. Most of the new NHS trusts which are based in the community see advantages in sending the patients presently treated in hospital, to receive their diagnostic work up and therapy in the community. I have mentioned that the trend for curative work has been moving away from super-specialists and surgeons towards the physicians and general practitioners. A further move towards hospital at home schemes is part of this trend.

The early hospitals at home were intended to back up inpatient care, thus allowing earlier discharge from hospital. In the USA, seven out of 10 hospitals have now developed such follow-up services, organized in a variety of ways. One of the main purposes of such schemes has been to reduce the likelihood of unplanned readmissions to hospital after patients have been discharged. Such readmissions are costly and undermine the ability of the hospital to plan its future workload. Such approaches also allow the hospitals to reduce the length of stay of patients. Many of the insurance systems in the USA now cover this form of care [213] as the companies realize the financial advantages of such an arrangement.

A number of US companies now provide financing for monitoring, giving nutrient solutions, appliances and such like for people in their own homes. This appears to have considerable commercial benefit for the insurance firms paying for the care and this in itself may promote further development. There can, on occasion, be some difficulty with developing such services in the UK, where community health staff, who are mainly nurses used to having a great deal of autonomy, may clash with specialist staff when they work in the community.

Increasingly, in the USA, home help agencies are being set up by hospitals as departments within the hospital. This has the advantage that such departments have to meet the quality and other requirements which are part of the US hospital accreditation system. It also makes it possible to have close liaison between the inpatient and home sectors. In particular, such things as record keeping and the control of treatment can be common to both hospital and the community. However, when moving from the hospital to the community, patients must also, at some point, move from secondary to primary care. The crossing of this administrative barrier, as with all interfaces, has the potential for losing information and therefore poses considerable problems in most health services.

Some remarkable community based hospital back up services have been developed. Marks [214] has recently described the South Hills Health System Home and Health Agency which is the largest home help agency in the USA [215]. It was established in Pittsburgh in 1963 and serves nine hospitals treating an average of 3000 patients each day. It employs over 300 staff, nurses, therapists and health care aides. Its services cover psychiatric, paediatric, physiotherapy, occupational therapy, speech therapy, social work and home help aid care. Health education supports the services and nutritional advice is available. It can provide care at home at virtually any level, including intravenous antibiotic therapy and nutritional care. It includes the use of life support machines.

The services are planned on a geographical basis. The team helps to develop discharge plans for patients in hospital and coordinate services, making sure that equipment is available and staff are ready to produce and amend care plans. A member of the team attends discharge planning rounds on each nursing unit within the hospitals in the system and visits the patient at home within 48 hours. The system is expensive, except in comparison with the cost of inpatient beds, so that so long as it is reducing length of stay it is cost effective. There is a temptation for such services to be even less aware of the importance of discharging patients than hospitals, in which case the overall costs can rapidly mount up.

It may be thought, at first sight, that such a system is simply the USA discovering the UK community health care system rather late in the day. However, such services seem to be better organized, coordinated and, in particular, targeted than most of such services in the UK. The USA service described is, of course, a flagship service, uniquely well organized and funded for that country, so it may be unfair to compare it with an overall service in the UK. However, such services are expanding and they appear to be developing as a standard approach. The system of payment for the service, through the large insurance companies, suggests that they, at any rate, are convinced of the cost benefits of such a service.

Most UK health authorities would have available some, but not all, of the services in the South Hills Agency. In particular, the close integration with hospital care is still a dream for most areas of the UK. A succession of other experiments has been set up where acute curative care is offered entirely outside the hospital, especially in Canada [216]. A number of such hospital at home schemes have also been set up in the UK. These are increasing rapidly in number, each with its own characteristics. In Seaton in Devon, a scheme has been set up to provide care for dependent elderly people. This includes the care of people with stroke, cancer and other diseases. It aims to provide acute care over the short term.

Perhaps the best known UK scheme has been running in Peterborough for some years [217]. It treats at home patients who would otherwise be admitted to hospital, either by completely preventing admission, or by taking people after an early discharge. At first the scheme employed nurses and unqualified aides separately from the community health services, therapists and social workers. Possibly because of this separateness the service was not at all well accepted by general practitioners. There were also difficulties between the hospital at home nurses and the existing community staff. Such free-standing schemes often have difficulty liaising with existing services. They are frequently set up using research money and are therefore required to be autonomous so that their effectiveness can be monitored. This, in itself, often makes them ineffective in a situation where good liaison with existing services is likely to be crucial to the success of the scheme.

It is not easy to avoid such problems, for, if the scheme is well integrated from the start, it is virtually impossible either to evaluate its effectiveness or, if it is thought to be ineffective, to close down the service later. In particular it is difficult to organize a control scheme where the traditionally organized service is not contaminated by the ideas being engendered by the new one. It is especially difficult to set up a randomized controlled trial to test the effectiveness of such services, for the professionals involved will be aware of and have an opinion on the likely effectiveness of the new method of working. This is likely to affect the way that they work and either undermine the new, untried service or undermine the old, discarded one.

The Peterborough scheme, after an initial phase in which the service was separately organized and funded, later became integrated into the general primary health care and community nursing services and now admits up to 400 patients per year. They are mainly suffering from stroke, cancer, hip fractures and elective hip and knee replacements. In addition, children on traction with congenital dislocation of the hip or fractured femurs are also being nursed at home [217]. However, as in the Seaton service, the main users of the service are elderly people with terminal disease or those who require intensive rehabilitation.

The authors who describe the Peterborough scheme suggest that such schemes need to be quite big to work effectively. One way around this might be not to rely on separate physiotherapists and occupational therapists for instance, who are expensive and a small number of whom go a long way, but to take on staff who are capable of performing both types of therapy, or of using mainly aides overseen by fully qualified staff seconded for a small number of sessions. Such changes in approach have important implications for training community care staff; this will be discussed in more detail in Chapter 11.

A randomized controlled trial of the Peterborough scheme was set up but the randomization failed because of lack of support by the general practitioners in the area. Interestingly, once the hospital at home scheme had been well established, their main objection was that they did not wish the control group to be treated in hospital.

This contrasts with attempts to set up new home care schemes for people with coronary heart disease where the general practitioners were insistent that most cases should be treated in hospital. It appears that a new and untried service becomes the norm within about 5 years for UK general practitioners. There is also the possibility, of course, that elderly people with terminal and rehabilitative care are seen as more 'naturally' falling into a community care approach than young people with coronary heart disease. This probably means that general practitioners feel that community care is not as 'safe' as hospital care and that it is therefore not suitable for younger people.

Community care requires a different set of talents from those which are commonly available in hospital. In particular, there needs to be much more emphasis on a range of skills within each person and a close understanding of what other professionals have to offer. In the UK, at present, we get around this problem by employing mainly nurses in the community and getting them to undertake most of the tasks. In addition, a few tasks are carried out by doctors, some by therapists, some by social workers and some by untrained aides or family members.

It would be more sensible to have a 'generic professional' together with a 'generic aide' who could do all of the things required of them in the community setting, dividing the tasks into those which require a high degree of training and those which do not.

Setting up a hospital at home scheme

In the UK, more new hospital at home schemes are likely to be set up by community based health trusts who see them as a 'patient friendly' and cost effective way of caring for acutely ill patients when compared with the alternative of inpatient care. Some work has been done to show that patients prefer hospital at home to going into an institution, but there is a dearth of information about comparative costs in the UK. If, as seems likely, acute care can be provided in this way at a lower cost than traditional inpatient care, the community based trusts may attempt to capture this lucrative secondary care. The trusts are under some pressure to move away from their traditional primary care work because fundholding general practitioners are likely to find it preferable to employ their own primary care nurses and health visitors in future. In addition, social services have the duty and the money to carry out many of the more socially orientated health functions, such as bathing, giving out medicines and cutting the toenails of dependent people, traditionally done by the community health services.

There appears to be little doubt that developing a hospital at home is more cost effective than expanding or building a new general hospital [218], if such an option exists. What is not clear is whether hospital at home is cheaper than using pre-existing district general hospital premises. Because of the great variability of costs in the hospital sector it is desirable to set up cost effectiveness projects in each place, prior to opening a new hospital at home scheme. There are a number of points which need to be taken into account on each occasion if this is to be the case.

Choice of medical condition

Great care has to be exercised in the choice of condition for hospitals at home at this stage in their development. It would be sensible for a completely new scheme to look after any conditions which require low levels of technical, nursing and clinical monitoring, but this would depend on the type of service that is envisaged and the professional assistance that is available. Part of the process of deciding who should be cared for is to find out what skills are available to treat patients. This is not measured in terms of the failure of a particular organ which is diseased, but in terms of how much the patients can manage for themselves, their degree of dependency.

Patients

The mental abilities of patients, their degree of dependence on others and the availability of someone to look after, for example, intravenous therapy, must be assessed before the service can be set up. Some areas of care are particularly specialized, for example wound healing, also patients who have a great deal of pain need to be looked after by a team well versed in such care.

Patients themselves may feel vulnerable if they are treated at home. Some prefer the thought of being in a hospital ward with a large number of facilities available for them if the worst should happen. Hospital at home, while likely to provide better creature comforts and a familiar environment for patients, nevertheless puts a certain amount of onus on them to get involved in their own cure. This is likely to be a bonus for the speed of recovery but some patients prefer 'to leave it to the doctors and nurses'. They prefer a formal approach which does not require self analysis or much effort beyond forbearance. However, it is likely that such people will not fare particularly well in hospital, because an acute general ward is not always a therapeutic environment. Sometimes it seems like a madhouse.

The need for good and intensive training of patients in order to help them in their process of recovery is self evident when they are being treated at home. No one is forgotten in the side ward or in the corner at the end when they are in their own bedroom. The active involvement of patients is also an essential part of community and home care. It is a new approach to the treatment of acutely ill people and therefore patients do not have a great deal of knowledge about the processes involved and what is expected of them. For this reason some groups have an audiovisual programme and instruction manual for the use of patients, families and professionals.

The acute care of someone at home may not be more time consuming or demanding on their family than the acute care of a close relative in hospital, but it will require a different approach. They will find themselves taking a much more active and more rewarding part in the therapeutic procedures. Manuals used in hospital at home schemes may include an emergency plan, schedules of what is to be expected, times when doctors or nurses will visit the patient, and what is expected of relatives who may be involved in injecting medication, managing fluid intake or assisting with physiotherapy.

General acceptability

It is essential that the approach used and the things expected of patients, relatives and staff are acceptable to all of them. This contrasts with hospital care where, to some degree, the therapy comes 'steamrollered' and often without warning. Patients may be over optimistic about the extent to which their family is willing, or wishes to become involved. They also tend to be over enthusiastic about the abilities of their carers. This tendency can best be weighed up by including the family in all negotiations about who does what. Professionals also need to develop a sixth sense to assess whether relatives are being overburdened.

Patients in hospital are subservient to a large and frightening organization. They are therefore extremely unwilling to criticize that organization, unless particular care is taken to make it obvious to patients that what they say will be treated confidentially and that there is no contact between the person collecting the information and professionals who may later be treating them. There is in addition a more subtle pressure on patients. In most acute wards there is a tradition of nurses being extremely busy all of the time. This is often because of understaffing on acute wards compounded by an expectation that nurses are expected always to look busy. In my auxiliary nursing days, if there was no obvious pressing work to do, we would be 'found some', usually making swabs or cleaning out cupboards.

The tradition still dies hard in UK hospitals that nurses are expected to be constantly on the move and that junior doctors are constantly on call. As a result of this set up, patients often feel sorry for the staff they are most in contact with and are very appreciative of the work done for them. They are therefore reluctant to complain about even quite outrageous actions. This can, on occasion, lead to the peculiar situation where a well run reasonably relaxed ward will receive more complaints than one where frenetic activity is the norm.

The result of all this is that it is sometimes difficult to get a realistic view of how good the service actually is from the people who use it. There have, however, been what appear to be reasonably objective methods of obtaining information about patient acceptability, some of which are mentioned in Chapter 10. The other side of this coin is that patients treated at home, especially close to their families, may be much more critical of the therapy that is being given. Relatives are more likely to overhear exchanges between doctors or nurses and the patient. Bad humour and rudeness are therefore much more difficult to get away with.

Problems of assessing cost effectiveness

The best means of assessing the cost effectiveness of hospital at home services is by using a study group and comparing it with a control group using a randomized method of allocation to one or the other. It is important in this sort of study to look at the cost of running the service and the costs to all of those concerned – patients, their families and carers, and the community at large. This can be tricky because decisions have to be made about how one should measure the cost of, for instance, pressure on family members as a result of being disturbed in the night.

It has been suggested [219] that a proper analysis of the effective use of resources would involve measures of mortality, morbidity, disability, discontent and discomfort together with their economic, social and psychological effect. Perhaps not surprisingly few studies have been this good in the past. Randomization in particular can often be undermined by well meaning general practitioners, community nurses and others.

A good review of the effects of home care has been put together by Hedrick and Inui [220]. They state that the early studies were poor and that the majority of them were assessed by the people running the schemes who would naturally be biased. Hedrick and Inui looked at 12 home care programmes which had a reasonable research design. There were considerable problems with bringing these together but they tentatively suggested that home care programmes do not affect mortality rates nor increase the use of nursing homes. They may have increased the use of outpatient services. In some cases costs seem to be less than in others, but the cost of home care is never greater than that in hospital. Most of the studies they assessed referred to acute care for elderly people, rather than acute treatment for younger adults.

The radical approach that hospital at home typifies is often looked at askance by general practitioners and other staff. In some areas, hospital at home has been used as a back up after hospital discharge allowing considerably reduced lengths of stay. This has sometimes been used for patients with difficult problems, for example people needing rehabilitation after fixation of a fractured neck of femur [221]. Evaluation of this work has used case control studies in order to avoid the difficulty of persuading general practitioners that randomization can be carried out without detriment to patients.

Assessing total costs

The costs of treatment for acute care are highest in the period immediately after the onset of the acute episode of disease. Home care schemes which take patients early on are therefore likely to be more costly than those aimed at reducing hospital length of stay, or which take only patients who require rehabilitation. They also have the greatest opportunity for saving money.

Adler and co-workers [222] itemized the benefits of home care services for patients, their families and society at large. They measured such things as the effect of the care on the psychological state of patients and relatives and the concern which these people have when being more involved with their own care. They made the point that all of these are important when assessing the impact of the treatment. A study of families with very seriously ill children kept at home on respirators [223] found that four in 10 of the families had considerable costs, often causing serious financial problems. The authors suggested that in these cases the substitution of family nursing for professional nursing was an important means of producing savings for the health service.

It appeared from these studies that hospital at home may not be cheaper than hospital inpatient care. However, the evidence collected so far has been concentrated on rehabilitation, especially for elderly people, which is a reasonably cheap phase of inpatient care compared with the early acute phase of an illness. The potential for saving is greatest, as I have said before, for early treatment. Care at home does allow relatives a number of benefits which are difficult to quantify in financial terms, such as a better understanding of the disease process, with less over-protection of the patient. It also helps to transfer the skill of managing patients with diseases to the patients and their families. It seems likely that these experiments, from small beginnings, will develop and become more adventurous. It has been estimated that virtually all medical care, apart from the most intensive care, could already be carried out in the home [224].

SURGICAL CARE ON A DAY PATIENT BASIS

The proportion and types of surgical operations carried out in day units, in contrast to conventional care in a hospital ward is increasing steadily. Figure 7.2 shows the increasing number of patients operated on as day cases in England over the past 20 years.

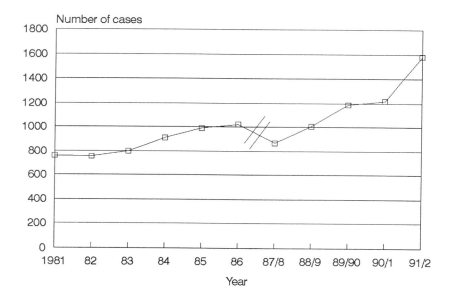

Figure 7.2 Day case admissions in England, 1981–1992. (The method of data collection changed between 1986 and 1987.)

The use of day surgery has spread to virtually all the specialties. Paediatric surgery in particular has taken to day care with great speed and commitment [225]. Some surgeons have gone so far as to suggest that virtually all minor and moderately complex surgery can be performed on a day basis with considerable financial savings. They suggest £105 saved per patient stay [226].

Others [227] have suggested that the expansion of day case surgery could largely clear the backlog of a number of operations with long waiting lists. An example is cataract operations which currently have a waiting list of about 50 000 patients in the UK. The authors of this paper suggest that the changes in the health service, where provider units who undertake more work get paid more, will find it very much in their interest to move almost entirely over to day surgery for this kind of operation. Curiously, a number of papers have suggested that with good liaison between hospital and the community an increase in routine day surgery has very little impact on the demand for general practitioner or community services [228], despite a large number of patients being discharged home on the same day as their operation.

It may be that for day surgery operative and anaesthetic methods have been adjusted to allow patients to get back to normal as quickly as possible. If this is the case, it is likely to have improved the outcome for patients, in terms of time off work and rehabilitation time. It may, of course, simply reflect the care with which patients are chosen for day surgery. It may be that those likely to have a difficult rehabilitation are admitted in the traditional manner so that those chosen for day surgery would not have needed follow-up community care, even if they had been admitted to hospital for a number of days.

Surgery is gradually giving way to medical care in a number of specialties. The treatment of peptic ulcer over the past 20 years has moved from being largely a surgical approach to a specialist medical treatment and is now becoming commonly treated in general practice. Recently, medication for the treatment of peptic ulcers has been released for sale without prescription in community pharmacies. This sort of change in therapy is likely to spread to the treatment of many other diseases, possibly with the back up of home computer based diagnostic programs, cutting out the need for the medical professionals.

Another example of the move from surgery to medicine is likely in the treatment of cancers. Developments in immunological control will allow specific treatment to be given to destroy abnormal cells using medical, rather than surgical techniques [229]. For other diseases, especially those caused by some inborn error, such as diabetes, gene therapy is likely to be important in cutting down the long term reliance on specialist help.

TREATING ACUTE MENTAL ILLNESS IN THE COMMUNITY

There is general agreement that most long term and rehabilitative psychiatric care can successfully be given to patients in the community if the service is well set up and responsive to the needs of the more complicated patients. Localized day hospitals and day centres for mentally ill people can, with a little imagination, be useful to a wide range of patients and give them support with financial, housing and other problems. They may even assist them in obtaining work, probably the most positive breakthrough that mentally ill people can achieve, in order to give them confidence and a feeling of acceptance by society.

There is increasing agreement about the possibility of treating even acutely mentally ill people in their own homes. Interestingly this, the most controversial area for home treatment, is also better researched than the management of more chronically ill patients. There appears to be an assumption that long term care or rehabilitation is best given locally without having to test the idea critically using randomized controlled trials and other research methods.

A number of papers, well summarized in a recent editorial [230], have reported trials comparing acute home and hospital based care for adult patients. Most of the services set up offer 'crisis intervention' provided by a mobile team. Work in the USA [231] showed that patients assessed and treated by a multidisciplinary team at home resulted in the home treated group having better social functioning, satisfaction, employment and drug compliance. Their use of inpatient beds fell [232]. A similar study in Australia also showed that home treatment was more effective and claimed that it was considerably cheaper than inpatient care with outpatient follow-up. Others, however, have suggested that the gains made in the early days are not sustained in the long term [233].

In the UK, several recent studies have compared home treatment with inpatient care. In one of these [234] about a third of the home care group required admission at some point. A 3-year randomized controlled trial held in London [235] showed that the home treatment group did require some time in hospital but this was about one-fifth as long as in the hospitalized group. A further study [236] showed that over a 1-year period home based treatment was more cost effective than inpatient care.

All of these studies agree that patients much prefer the home based system. These systems are generally more acceptable both to patients and relatives. Patients seem to come out of them particularly well with regard to their social functioning. However, the more closely one looks at costs, the less the difference between the two services appears to be. My own experience in this area suggests that the inpatient model may be a little cheaper, but, because patients get lost and are then readmitted as an emergency, costs are increased. The overall costs are therefore roughly the same but fewer patients have to go through the damaging process of being readmitted when their ability to cope in the community breaks down. There is still a need for small inpatient units in the locality, possibly near to the day hospital or the day centre, but these will be considerably smaller than inpatient facilities have been and considerably smaller than they are now.

NO LONGER TIED TO HOSPITAL: LABORATORY SERVICES

Laboratory work is an important part of the specialization of acute health care and health services. Close access to laboratories which can assist with diagnostic scientific data is often given as a reason for admitting a patient to hospital. The laboratory based departments have traditionally been brought together in the major hospitals in the UK. The reason for this has been that many diseases or conditions have similar pathological changes and therefore require similar tests. On the other hand, a series of different tests may be done using similar techniques with modern autoanalysers which, simply by changing the reagents, can measure a number of different things.

Hospital laboratories were originally placed where they are in order to bring together a very specialized workforce. The technicians were experts in the particular skills required for examining fluids or blood cells or, for example, slides taken from cancerous tissue in the operating theatre. Much of the work that the skilled technicians have done in the past is now being performed by machinery which requires only to be operated.

A more recent change is that general practitioners in charge of their own budget for their non-emergency hospital work, will not have the incentive to refer patients to hospital in order to have straightforward pathological tests performed. Until about 1980, general practitioners could often not even request tests. They had to refer patients to specialists in hospital who would then order the tests. There was therefore an incentive for them, as the hospital laboratory services were free, not to perform any tests of their own but to send patients for testing to hospital. In the future, general practitioners are likely to use laboratory facilities which do not carry hospital overheads. Such stand alone laboratories run by private companies are beginning to develop in the UK.

Possibly because of this referral system from general practitioners to specialists, UK doctors do not use a great number of tests compared with their foreign counterparts. They tend to rely heavily on the history, symptoms and signs of disease. Because of this the laboratory service is also reasonably cheap in the UK compared with other countries. There has therefore not been a great deal of pressure on laboratories to cut their costs by enlarging. In North America some centralized laboratories are extremely large. Indeed the largest is 30 times larger than the biggest NHS laboratory. Such a system can provide considerable savings and, because of its good organization and communications provides rapid turn around times.

A number of new technological developments are likely to bring about changes in the way that these laboratories are organized. The first of these is the advent of freely available computers and data processing. The rapid transfer of large quantities of information and the production of new methods of measurement make analysis relatively simple and relatively independent of the place where the sample is taken. Some of the new techniques mentioned in Chapter 4, such as the use of highly specific antibodies to detect abnormal tissues in different diseases, can often be used as kits in the doctor's office. However, their production is so specialized that very few hospital laboratories produce their own. The existence of the hospital laboratory, both for carrying out tests and as a convenient local centre, is therefore threatened.

New changes within the UK, particularly the requirement for provider units to decide on the costs of the processes they undertake, means that the trusts will look in detail at the cost of each procedure. Unnecessary laboratory costs will be an obvious area where cutbacks may be brought about. Comparisons between different trusts will be made obvious by the contracting system.

The Audit Commission surveyed laboratories in 1990 and showed the average laboratory processed 70 000 samples in a year with five staff. In 1992, a laboratory has shown that it can process 300 000 samples with 2.75 staff. This underlines the extremely rapid change going on in laboratory work. It will be possible to perform some of the urgent complex analyses at ward level or in clinics using kits. It may well be that general practitioners will use a central laboratory service as it will prove to be cheaper and probably capable of a more rapid response than hospital based laboratories.

Some services pathologists perform cannot be automated. One is the need to perform post-mortems, though this again might be more effectively done at some central point rather than in individual hospitals. There is a need for better facilities for post-mortem work in many hospitals in the UK. There is also the need for more specialist knowledge away from teaching centres, particularly in such areas as paediatric and forensic pathology. The latter is already largely centralized to overcome this lack of expertise.

CHANGES TO THE EXISTING SPECIALTIES

Programme groups are increasingly working across the present specialty boundaries. These programmes work on cancer treatment, cardiovascular disease and gastroenterology. It seems likely that these groups will increasingly form specialist teams with preventive, primary care and secondary care becoming amalgamated. Some moves in this direction, especially with the development of specialist community nurses, have been seen for the treatment of some complex diseases such as diabetes or epilepsy, and of specific problems such as the treatment of incontinence. Such moves are likely to expand rapidly over the next few years, if only because purchasers of health services will tend to purchase that way. The pressure for providers to try to provide an integrated service in the same way is likely to be great.

Effects of changes: rehabilitation and long term care

8

REDUCING CHRONIC DISEASE WITH GENETIC DIAGNOSIS

Changes that are occurring in genetics will have an impact on the number of people with some chronic diseases and the disability that they cause. The usefulness of most genetic diagnostic methods has yet to be proved. Genetic diagnosis is not a single approach, there are several different technological aspects to it. The relationship between a genetic abnormality in the nucleus of a cell and the disease it causes is not a simple one. The genetic makeup of a person interacts with the environment in which he or she lives so that quite marked genetic changes may not cause an individual to be badly affected by the genetic defect. Most diseases associated with genetic change have a number of different sets of abnormal genes. In the case of cystic fibrosis there are hundreds of different genetic changes associated with the one disease process.

A major difficulty with screening unaffected populations for genetic abnormalities is that the genetic changes detected may not ultimately result in the typical disease or the disease may be only a minor affliction. This becomes particularly important if prenatal screening shows genetic abnormalities. There may be a temptation to abort a foetus because of genetic abnormalities that might not have resulted in the person being disabled.

Even where the likely outcome is known to be bad there are problems about giving people information about their genetic makeup. Such problems are already seen in families who have a rare fatal disease, Huntington's chorea, which shows itself late in life. Psychological abnormalities may result from the threat of the disease where there is a 50% chance of the individual suffering from it in later life. It can be imagined that information that one definitely has the abnormal genetic component and that one will therefore be extremely likely to die of Huntington's chorea will cause even more psychological upset to these families.

On the other hand, in future, it may be discovered that some common diseases, for example cancers or heart disease, may be particularly prevalent in groups of people with particular mixtures of genetic material. It may be, for instance, that certain genetic changes make some individuals who smoke at very high risk from lung cancer. If it were possible to identify these individuals early on, it might be that particular attention could be given to them to encourage them to avoid smoking cigarettes. Such preventive work would, of course, help to prolong the life of those individuals.

EARLY TREATMENT MEANS FASTER REHABILITATION

Patients receiving acute medical and surgical care are spending less and less time under that care. They are being discharged from hospitals or day units increasingly quickly. There have been worries that this rapid turn around would put considerable demands on the existing community services in helping people to get back to normal. I have mentioned that this does not seem to be the case when the possibility has been studied [237]. Reasonably fit people of all ages who come into hospital for a brief spell, be it day surgery, keyhole surgery or the treatment of a single medical condition, appear to manage to rehabilitate themselves reasonably well.

The cost to families of looking after the patient when he or she returns from day surgery appears to be balanced by the cost of visiting and providing extra night clothing and other things for patients staying in hospital for some days [238]. Day patients do not seem to need the backup facilities that are essential for mentally ill or elderly people, who are already commonly rehabilitated in the community.

People using day services do not appear to need formal rehabilitation, in contrast to a proportion of people admitted as inpatients. It may be that a long stay in hospital, of itself, is damaging, so that the reduced length of stay also reduces the need for a recovery period. It is certainly the case that the less invasive surgery that allows for shorter stays is also easier to recover from. But there is an additional point. Hospitals are quite dangerous places. Poor sleep, because of being awakened early and noisy general wards, poor food, over medication, especially overuse of night sedation, are all factors that exhaust patients.

ADVERSE EFFECTS OF HOSPITAL

The effect of hospitals themselves may increase the need for rehabilitation. Elderly people in particular seem to suffer as a result of being admitted to hospital. There can often be complications unrelated to the problem which caused their original admission [239]. In particular, bed rest can cause reduced blood volume, bone loss, less efficient heart beats and sensory deprivation. These can cause an older person to go into a state of irreversible decline. The effects can be avoided by modifying the usual acute hospital environment, avoiding bed rest where possible, helping elderly people to get together to talk and avoiding such things as the traditional high hospital bed, noise at night and alterations to patients' normal pattern of sleep and waking.

A number of diseases are very commonly associated with admission to hospital. Cancer patients can be badly affected by loss of function of their limbs due to peripheral nerve damage and other symptoms caused by drugs for the treatment of their cancer [240]. A particularly severe form of hospital induced illness has been called 'cascade iatrogenesis'. It is defined as a sequence of adverse events triggered by an initial medical intervention [241]. It is, as might be expected, most common in elderly patients, those who were most impaired on admission and those with the most severe forms of disease. This is presumably because these groups react most adversely to therapy and are also most likely to receive the most aggressive treatment.

Some authors have described a method of collecting adverse patient occurrences in hospital [242]. A study from the University Hospital in Maastricht in The Netherlands has also shown that age, length of stay and diagnostic group are closely related to adverse occurrences. Some operations, particularly malignant disorders of the ear, nose and throat, are likely to be associated with adverse patient occurrences and the study suggested that particular care should be given to these patients.

In acute general inpatient surgery, sepsis can be a considerable problem [243]. There is a marked variation in the type of patient most affected by sepsis; the worst affected appear to be different in different areas. Some people have suggested that this variation is because of pockets of bad practice and that local studies can identify units or surgeons who seem to get high rates of sepsis in their patients. This may be a useful way of pinpointing units or wards which are giving a poor quality service.

The longer patients stay in hospital the more likely they are to have complications brought on by the hospital regime itself. One study of patients kept in hospital for more than 15 days showed that almost two-thirds of the patients had at least one complication caused by the admission, half of which were thought to be preventable [244]. Patients in intensive care units are not safe from such complications. Ferraris and Propp suggested that one doctor-induced drug complication occurred in a third of all patients [245]. These complications were much more likely to occur if patients were in intensive care for more than 72 hours. Even the uniforms worn by staff have been found to have adverse effects on the mental state of some patients [246]. The presence of hospital induced complications does not, in itself, guarantee that a community based alternative will be better. It does suggest, however that hospitals are not entirely safe, even without the effect of the illness.

REHABILITATION AT HOME: AN EFFECTIVE OPTION

In a study of 200 patients, Fraser [247] showed, in a comparison between patients treated at home and those treated in a hospital physiotherapy department, that the improvement in their physical condition was about the same. Costs were also virtually identical for the treatments given, if ambulance costs were omitted. By adding ambulance costs, the hospital based physiotherapy treatment was three times as expensive as that given at home. Patients treated at home seemed to require less treatment time to give similar results. This is because therapists spend time guiding and training relatives and other people caring for patients so that they understand the disease suffered by the patients and the best way to help them to improve. This study suggested that the amount of time spent travelling to and from hospital in an ambulance, the amount of time waiting for it, together with a one in five chance of having the journey cancelled without warning, has a very poor effect on patients visiting the hospital outpatient department.

The attitude of the family to the rehabilitation of patients after they get home is very important. This was confirmed accidentally in an experimental study which compared two groups of patients who had had strokes [248]. The first of these was treated in a stroke unit, the second in a normal ward in hospital. Patients who were treated in the stroke unit showed a greater improvement in their ability to perform normal activities when they were discharged home compared with those who had been in a ward.

The part of the study relevant to my argument was at the conclusion of the formal part. The authors found that patients who had been treated in the stroke unit were more likely, if independent when they left the unit, to relapse into dependence on their family for the activities they needed such as bathing themselves and cooking over the following year, in contrast to those who had been in a normal ward (Figure 8.1). Those who were dependent on others when they were sent home from the unit were less likely to become independent after they arrived home.

The authors of the study suggested that the deterioration in the patients who had shown an initial improvement in the stroke unit was due to their relatives being careful with patients who had been in the new, rather imposing, stroke unit. The specialist and high tech atmosphere of the unit suggested to the relatives that the patients treated there had been very ill and therefore needed to be carefully looked after compared with people in an ordinary hospital ward. The relatives therefore appeared to be more protective of those patients when they arrived home, reversing their improvement.

It is likely that any hospital admission, compared with looking after a patient at home, is likely to have a similar impression on relatives. This may be one reason why most good trials comparing the home or hospital treatment of patients needing rehabilitation show either no advantage either way, or an advantage for the home care approach. This is despite better access to various forms of apparatus and to therapists in hospital.

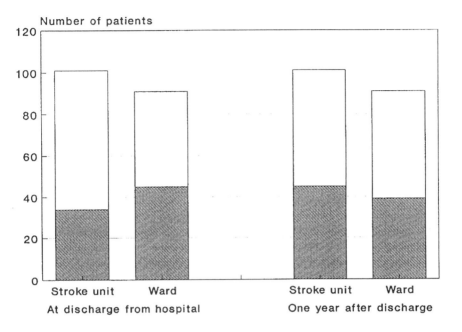

Figure 8.1 Patients treated initially in a stroke unit were most likely to be dependent on others (shaded) than independent (unshaded) at one year. Reproduced with permission from [248].

Hospital, by its very complexity and strangeness, may suggest to relatives that, after discharge, patients need careful handling, thus maintaining the sick role of the patient and delaying a return to normal life. This may be due, as much as anything, to the absence of the patient from the daily home routine for a period.

Health services in leisure or shopping centres

Rehabilitation is moving out into the community. The new found confidence developed by social services, for providing locally based services as a result of the Community Care Act, together with their contacts with private, voluntary groups and community based health trusts is leading them to provide a wide range of services, often with an emphasis on improving or delaying disability. Many social services departments have waited long and patiently for health services, especially physiotherapy and occupational therapy services, to move into the day centres, and residential homes, so that their disabled clients can receive local physical maintenance therapy, rather than having to deteriorate completely before being sent off to the local hospital. It has happened, but only rarely. Now, with a small amount of energy, social services can buy in their own therapists to assist people who are recovering from disease to get back to full fitness.

In future, it is likely that people who have been ill will take part in more general community fitness activities to maintain the progress that they have made. A person who has eaten too much over Christmas and wants to get rid of some excess weight, a mother who has recently had a baby and wants to tone up her muscles, a man who has had a mild heart attack, or a woman of 70 who has had a mild stroke, all have similar needs for a range of graduated exercises. The community has such facilities available for the first two of these in non-health facilities. It seems sensible to combine the needs of all four types of people with aerobic exercises and swimming in the local leisure facilities, rather than making them travel away from home and wait hours for a 20 minute session with a physiotherapist helper.

It can only be a matter of time before private gymnasiums in the UK move away from trying to produce heavyweight champion boxers, or making slim sexy people even more slim and sexy, and realize that health promotion can be big business locally. Those who are relatively fat, poor or elderly form the majority of the population and have the greatest needs, if only the market can be captured. People needing more intensive therapy will receive this in their own homes, where relatives can assist and the care given will be customized to the needs of that patient, living in that house, and hoping to get back to his or her specific job.

PROBLEMS WITH EVALUATING REHABILITATION

Rehabilitation services abound with old wives' tales and untested fads. There are a number of reasons for this. Progress in rehabilitation is quite difficult to measure. It is essentially about changes in disability and handicap which have not been popular measures in health orientated work until recently. Even now, the use of such measures tends to be restricted to specialists in rehabilitation. The medical profession have been very slow to pick up their use. One exception recently has been the suggestion by the British Geriatric Society that all patients admitted to geriatric wards should, on admission and discharge, receive an activities of daily living measure [249].

A further problem is that rehabilitation is needed when a cure has not been immediately or fully effective. There is therefore a tendency to believe (sometimes rightly) that the traditional medical service has failed. Doctors are very bad at admitting failure or dealing with patients whose treatment has not worked. The patients therefore tend to be frustrated and confused, often feeling abandoned by conventional medicine. This leaves the stage clear for the unconventional, sometimes the charlatan.

Another problem has been the fragmentation of expertise in rehabilitation. By definition, much of the success of rehabilitation, particularly in patients with relatively long term problems, has been to do with their psychological and social adaptation before they can get back to normality or some stable state. The divisions of the professions, notably those between medicine and social work, and within medicine the separation of psychiatry, psychology, speech therapy, occupational therapy and physiotherapy from each other and from medicine and nursing, has meant that it is often difficult to organize a comprehensive service that is not extremely expensive or very fragmented.

A few attempts have been made to develop 'team training' in order to bring together and coordinate the expertise of these groups, but to date each of the separate members of the team have been educated separately, both at under-graduate and graduate level. These factors have all delayed the development of rehabilitation anywhere, including in the community, despite the fact that such developments make sense, bring patients nearer to a normal environment, and are likely to be preferred by most patients.

HOME REHABILITATION AND SELF HELP GROUPS

I have already mentioned that an important development in community based rehabilitation has been the tendency for people to be given more control over their own care. A number of projects have been set up that have taken these ideas further. The large number relating to different diseases suggests that virtu-ally all other chronic disease problems could be approached similarly. A good example of such a method of rehabilitation was examined by Lorig and co-authors [250]. This was a comparison of 100 patients with arthritis, some of whom were given a self management course for the control of their symptoms. They were randomly allocated into three groups, one group taught by lay people, the second by professionals and the third not given a self management course.

Arthritis, which is a common disease with relatively few specialist profes-sionals available, is particularly well placed for the use of lay teaching. The arthritis self management course taught patients an overview of arthritis and its types, some exercises for relaxation, guidance on the use of medicines, nutri-tional advice and methods of solving a number of problems encountered in daily living. There were sessions on the prevention of damage to and the protec-tion of joints and an evaluation of alternative therapies. The sessions concluded with techniques for obtaining information from physicians and others involved with the treatment.

This study [250] showed that participants in the courses taught by lay leaders showed a considerable increase in their knowledge, the amount of exercise they took and the degree of relaxation they were able to exhibit. There was also a considerable decrease in the disability suffered by the patients over the time that the training was given. Similar changes were seen with the professionally led groups. The patients who received no assistance in helping them to cope with their disabilities, other than conventional therapy, showed no particular improvements or deterioration during the time of the study.

There was relatively little difference between the lay and the professionally led groups in most of the measures mentioned except that those in the professionally led group had a greater increase in their knowledge of their disease than those led by the lay people. In contrast, those led by lay people were better at relaxation than those led by professionals. The lay courses attracted a higher number of those invited than the professional courses.

This was a small study but on an extremely important subject. Other groups have used lay people as providers of health education. The Reach to Recovery programme of the American Cancer Society has one course in which women who have had mastectomies visit new mastectomy patients in hospital. Other lay groups have been used for sex education [251], for teaching the elderly about community health [252], and helping people to cope with depression [253] and incontinence [254].

The use of lay people as instructors has a number of important advantages for the rehabilitation of patients. People who have a direct knowledge of a problem, either because they suffer from it or because they have relatives who do, are more likely to be successful in changing the behaviour of other patients. This has been suggested by theoretical work [255, 256] and has been confirmed practically in several large health education programmes [251, 257]. The potency of lay people to be more persuasive when trying to change behaviour is often overlooked. The greatest benefits of using lay people as instructors are often perceived to be the fact that they form a large pool of available people and that they are likely to be cheaper than using professionals.

Many of these studies, interesting though they are, have not attempted to be particularly critical in their evaluation of the work that they do, nor have they tried to cost the interventions. An exception to this was reported by Bergner and co-workers [258]. This was a randomized controlled trial to decide on the effectiveness and cost of home nursing care for patients with chronic lung disease. This approach was compared with regular visits by home care nurses without special respiratory skills and with another group that did not receive such home care. The authors suggest that many people are convinced that there are circumstances in which home care can delay or prevent admission to hospital and that home care is better for caring for or curing people with chronic disease. Examples of such home care programmes have been around for over 40 years [259].

The Bergner *et al.* study repays a more detailed look. The disease in question, chronic obstructive pulmonary disease, is a major health problem. The effects of the disease on the function of patients are extreme, the majority of patients have a mixture of chronic bronchitis and emphysema. Patients who are severely affected are likely to have a life expectancy of considerably less than 5 years. A number of specialist approaches have been used to help people with such pulmonary disease, particularly the use of drugs, chest percussion to get rid of secretions, and sometimes drainage. The early treatment of acute infections with antibiotics is important, as is training in breathing techniques. Others have tried exercise therapy. Psychosocial support with individual and family counselling and preventive therapy through advice on stopping smoking and reducing occupational exposure to irritants are also important.

The disease therefore requires a complex approach. Previous studies have been disappointing in that the disease appears to progress as rapidly no matter what the therapy. Patients do seem to get some benefit in terms of their well-being and ability to carry out their normal activities over the short term if the complex regime is followed. The Bergner *et al.* study was therefore set up to compare how well patients complied with the regime if specialist respiratory home care nurses or non-specialist home care nurses treated the patients. The study was important, firstly because it was a randomized trial and was therefore unlikely to reach its findings by chance or the bias of the therapists, and secondly because it showed the possibilities of using specialist nurses in the community and carefully costed those services.

Figure 8.2 shows a comparison between disability score at 6 months and 1 year. There was no difference in survival between the different groups. There was a slight advantage in ability, both at 6 months and 1 year, for the group receiving special nursing care.

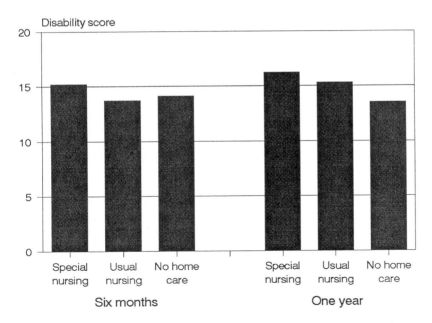

Figure 8.2 Special nursing care resulted in slightly better levels of ability than home nursing. (Reproduced with permission from [258].)

The mean total health care costs between the different groups are shown in Figure 8.3. The specialist respiratory home care group consistently cost more than either of the other two groups. It seems therefore that giving special services to unselected patients at home marginally improves their health but costs a great deal more. This was largely because the specialist home nurses visited more often and made more phone calls than the standard home care nurses.

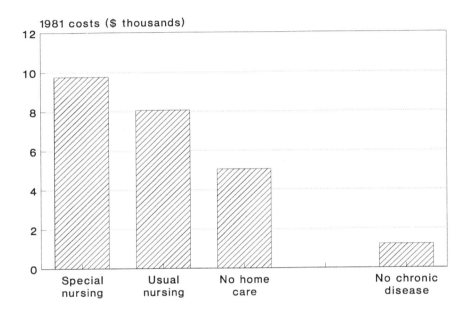

Figure 8.3 Costs of managing chronic lung disease. (Reproduced with permission from [258].)

In 1982, the United States General Accounting Office reviewed home care demonstrations for Medicare patients over the previous 8 years. None of the demonstrations [260] found that the cost of care for chronically ill patients was increased or reduced among those that used home care compared with those that were treated in hospital. There was no effect on physical or mental function in most of the studies, though one showed an improvement for home care. A number of assessments of elderly people and their care at home have shown changes in longevity but fewer have shown changes in their disability ratings. A meta-analysis of such studies concluded that there was benefit to be obtained from home care for elderly people, though these studies did not contain costing data [261]. It appears possible from this analysis that it is easier to prevent death than to reduce the amount of disability suffered by chronically ill people.

THE OTHER EXTREME: THE CASE OF ORTHOPAEDICS

One of the difficulties of giving a boost to rehabilitation services has been the extraordinary lack of enthusiasm shown by some specialists for rehabilitation in any of its forms. It has been mentioned that the rehabilitation services have been slow to develop as a specialty in their own right. This is usually because the other specialties have claimed that they are expert in a particular set of diseases and therefore only they can oversee the necessary physical or mental changes required for ensuring a full recovery.

An exception to this is the care of elderly women with fractured necks of femur. Orthopaedic surgeons who may claim a god-like expertise when faced with any other problem have often given in when faced with an old woman who is a bit slow getting out of bed and, in the UK, have tended to call in geriatricians to help. How a subspecialty so given to pride can suddenly become dependent on other colleagues of lower status is difficult to say.

The so called orthogeriatric unit is the result. These units have become very popular, despite an early randomized trial which showed them to be costly and ineffective [262], and further trials which were equivocal [263, 264]. They seem to me to be a good example of an answer to a doctor's problem, rather than a patient's problem. The orthopaedic surgeons continue to be unable to organize a reasonable service for such people despite such help [265].

LONG TERM CARE: PURCHASING COMMUNITY SERVICES

The problem with long term residential care is that everyone sees him- or herself as being on the shores of the Styx, either as boatman or passenger [266]. This depressing approach to long term care appears to have dominated the health service since the days of the workhouse infirmary and may have been one of the reasons behind the recent impetus to move the whole area out of the hospital, indeed the health sector, as rapidly as possible. Another reason may be cost. Whatever the motives, the move into small homely units in the community is to be welcomed. There appears to be a feeling that small, homely places do not belong in the health service, a myth that I hope this book will help to dispel. Whoever runs these units will have much to do to ensure that the quality of the services given and the financial burden on patients is contained.

I mentioned in Chapter 2 that there may or may not be a rise in the number of people, especially elderly people, with long term diseases. However, the numbers are not likely to drop much, if at all. The need for long term care is therefore likely to continue. In my opinion, many long stay wards remaining in the health service at present are a disgrace. Change is certainly required. Stimulated by the recent changes in the structure of the health service a number of health authorities have looked closely at the way they care for people with long term problems. Some have used more imagination than in the past. Sadly this difference in approach, generally away from hospital care and into a series of different options, was not led by a feeling of dissatisfaction with the existing service but by financial and quality measures imposed on the health authorities, especially by the NHS and Community Care Act [267]. This has led health services to examine what they should and should not do and in addition what they do well and what they do badly.

Long term care in the health service has been much affected by changes in social services provision of residential homes and the development of private residential and nursing homes. A period of economic decline in the mid 1970s led to a reduction in the money available to local authorities. This hit voluntary organizations, who are partly dependent on local authorities (not, as is sometimes assumed, totally dependent on volunteers or voluntary contributions) for money to produce most of their services. They, in turn, persuaded local social security officers to pay financial benefits to elderly and disabled people in residential homes if those people were unable to afford their own fees.

This arrangement was legalized in 1983 by the Conservative government. One-third of pensioners were already receiving supplementary pension and this automatically entitled them, as long they had less than £3000 in capital, to obtain support for admission to a private residential or nursing home. Voluntary organizations had originally led the campaign for this new source of money, but the main winners since then have been the owners of private residential and nursing homes for old people. The move was assisted by geriatricians whose long term hospital beds had been under increasing pressure as the acute care of elderly people moved into the general hospitals in the 1970s.

Figure 8.4 shows the growth of private and voluntary residential homes from 1968 to 1990 that sprang from these changes in the law. The increase in private and voluntary nursing homes occurred in concert with a lesser, but definite reduction in the number of local authority residential homes and NHS long term hospital places [268].

Long term nursing care became effectively free on demand for about a third of elderly people no matter whether they were disabled or not. It worked out that about two-thirds of those who applied came out of hospital beds. Despite this, the take up of places was not very great. It appears that chronically ill people in the UK enter residential or nursing homes only as a last resort.

The use of private residential and nursing homes increased mainly due to their increasing availability. Entrepreneurs, encouraged by high property prices and a potentially huge demand for the service, built more and more homes. The costs of such care to the government began to soar. The community care part of the NHS and Community Care Act was largely born out of the worries engendered by these soaring prices. It was designed to reduce the state subsidy

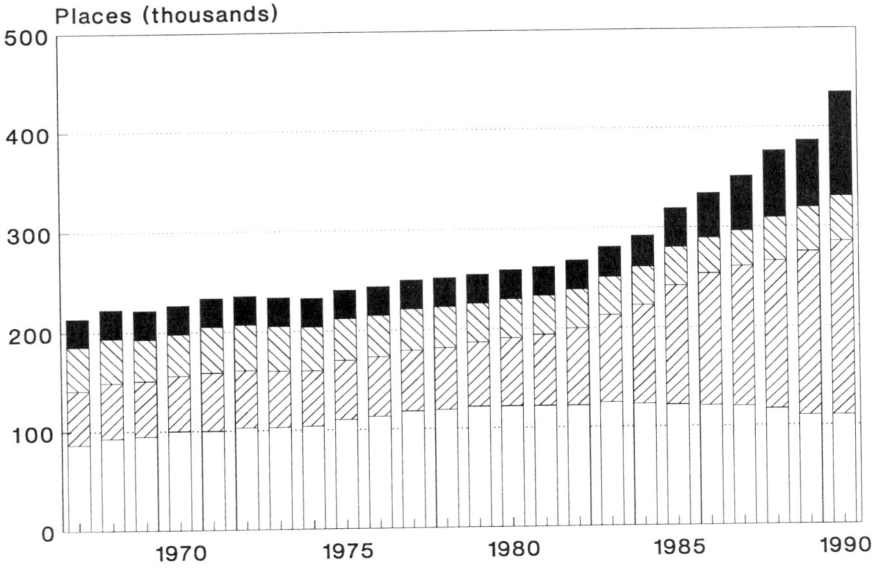

Figure 8.4 Nursing and residential care places in England. Private and voluntary nursing homes (■); NHS continuing care (▧); private and voluntary residential homes (▨); local authority residential homes (□). (Reproduced with permission from [268].)

of private long term care for poor people by bringing in a test of physical and mental fitness. People wanting financial help had to fail the test before they were given that help. The Act also transferred the money held by social security officers to social work departments.

Social work departments were also made responsible for carrying out the tests of fitness and the test of finances originally carried out by the social security departments. This at first proved quite a difficult job for social services and seemed to cause an initial delay in some areas for elderly people needing a decision, though this now seems to have sorted itself out [269].

The Act allows this transferred money, now held by social services, to be used to maintain people at home, instead of only being available to help maintain them in private residential or nursing homes. Early reports have been that about two-thirds of the people who would normally have gone into residential homes have opted to remain at home with assistance (about a third of those who might have been expected to go into nursing homes). Patients in acute hospital beds who needed long term health care had increasingly been using private nursing homes until the Community Care Act. Some long term care wards in hospitals still exist, but many of them are in poor physical condition with unpleasant physical layouts. They are particularly unsuitable for elderly people who are disabled and look similar to, and are often in the same buildings as, the workhouse infirmaries.

PRINCIPLES OF PURCHASING

The division of the health service into purchasers and providers, gives the opportunity for setting out the principles which should be used for purchasing such long term care instead of simply using what is available. A number of different groups have suggested principles which should be applied to the purchase of services. An example of such principles was laid down by the Welsh Health Planning Forum [270]:

- health gain focused (i.e. adding life to years and years to life)
- people centred
- resource effective.

It is a measure of the ephemeral nature of strategic planning principles that these have already been overturned by three others [271] but they appear to be only semantically different:

- ever improving health
- real choice for patients
- stewardship.

Health gain, or, in the new phrase, ever improving health, is the central guiding principle. The other two appear to be descriptions of how the improvement should be achieved. The idea of improving health also suggests that any chosen intervention should have the effects described to a significantly greater extent than doing nothing and to a greater extent than the next best treatment. These principles are very similar to those adopted originally by the WHO in its 'Health for All 2000' [272] movement. However, the WHO proposals include two further principles:

- adding equity to health
- adding health to life.

It is instructive as there is a rising concern about equity in all health services at present [273, 274], especially in the area of community care [275], to use all four.

The first problem for a health service purchaser is to decide whether the service should be part of the health service at all or whether some other organization should be providing the assistance. There is no definition of what is health care as distinct from social care [276]. This may be obvious for the difference between, say, a person with acute appendicitis and someone who is lonely, but there are a number of grey areas. Long term care for dependent people is one of them.

Long term care is mainly provided by relatives with no medical or nursing training and often with minimal assistance from health or other services. The degree of tending which such people require is of an intensity that only a devoted relative or relatives can provide. For groups of such people, high staffing and skill levels appear to be essential. Long term health care of groups of disabled people with an extreme degree of dependency can be very poor. Where performed properly it requires considerable skill in the care of their skin, bladder and bowels (traditionally nursing tasks) and providing company or assisting to keep the premises clean (definitely social tasks). Other types of care, such as maintaining mobility, assistance with personal cleanliness, cutting toenails and assistance with feeding are difficult to define as either nursing or social tasks. The combination of stimulating social care and good medical and nursing care is unusual.

Doctors with an interest in the field are few and far between and, in my experience, they are nearly always geriatricians or psychogeriatricians. As traditional leaders of the health professionals they can provide legitimacy to the job as many people are scornful of the skills needed for supporting good long term care. The features of this form of care are that it is a long term process of compromise, rather than being analytical. It is therefore at odds with the scientific mechanistic approach which some doctors believe to be at the heart of modern medicine.

Until recently, the combination of nurses, therapists and a highly motivated physician have only been found in hospital and therefore the service had to be in a hospital. This is no longer the case. Slowly, in a way akin to that seen for changes in paediatrics mentioned in Chapter 2, the emphasis of long term care of adults has gradually changed.

For long term care, a therapeutic approach that emphasizes the future potential of the person being treated and helps him or her to acquire new skills is likely to be more successful than replacing lost skills with another person or a machine to do the function instead (the prosthetic approach). Professor Grimley Evans is a strong advocate of the former [277]. He described an elderly woman who had some difficulty in getting to the shops to buy food. The answer to this problem, as prescribed by the professional who visited, was to ask meals on wheels to deliver meals five times a week. The elderly woman, being very grateful, did not like to refuse, so gave the food to her cat and continued with her lifetime hobby as a cordon bleu cook.

The therapeutic approach remains unusual in the health service, but has occasionally been allowed to develop in a medical setting or in one run by voluntary groups. An example of the success of such an approach, largely under the influence of health professionals, is in some branches of the hospice movement. If the approach is right, it does not matter where the therapy is being given or who manages it. However it does seem, from experience, more likely that the therapeutic approach will develop in the home of a patient, rather than in hospital.

HEALTH GAIN OR EVER IMPROVING HEALTH

Most people would agree that health has two components: extending life and extending the period of good quality life. These have been described, rather fancifully, by the WHO as adding years to life and life to years.

Adding years to life

The shores of the Styx may not seem the right place to be adding years to life. Figures on the survival of patients in different types of long term care are shown in Figure 8.5 [278].

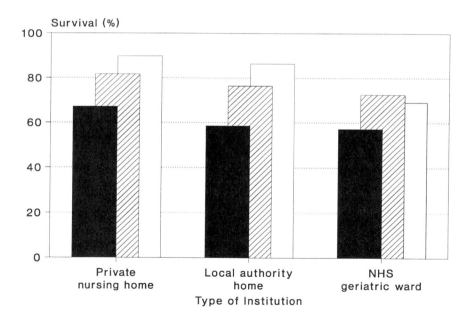

Figure 8.5 Survival of those with severe (solid shading), moderate (striped shading) and no (unshaded) disability is lowest in long term geriatric wards. Reproduced with permission from [278].

In order to make fair comparisons, the survival of patients was compared for those with different degrees of disability because some services deal with more disabled people, who would be expected to have a lower survival rate. Figure 8.5 shows that people at all levels of disability have a considerably better chance of surviving in a private nursing home than in an NHS long term geriatric ward.

There may be differences, even within the disability groups, in the severity of those in one form of residence compared with others. Nevertheless, a purchaser would need to be persuaded that it was not the poor environment in the geriatric hospital, with problems of cross-infection from chest complaints, or the generally depressing atmosphere of the place, which caused the excess death rate.

A small randomized controlled trial on the use of nursing homes run by the NHS showed, in contrast, that about a third of patients in the nursing home group died in a year compared with a quarter of those in a traditional long stay geriatric ward [279]. This finding was not statistically significant, for the numbers were small, and represented a relatively low mortality overall, but they give one pause for thought.

Adding life to years

Long term care at home has been compared with a hospital alternative, without using randomized controlled trials. One report, which studied 101 patients in Darlington, suggested that home care was better than long term hospital care overall [280]. The home care group had a higher death rate after 6 months, which reduced at 12 months, but the researchers said that a higher proportion of the home care patients were receiving care for terminal illness, which explained the difference. What a pity they did not randomize!

There was considerable advantage to the patients in the home care group in their well-being, compared with those who remained in hospital. Their degree of disability was the same in both places but a wide range of social activity levels were greater for the home care group (Figure 8.6).

The randomized trial by Bowling *et al.* [279], which compared an NHS nursing home and long stay geriatric wards, found that people going into the nursing home deteriorated more rapidly mentally and physically than those on the geriatric wards. The study had a number of flaws but, nevertheless, as a randomized trial it must give some pause to the wholehearted advocates of putting people into long term care in NHS nursing homes.

Adding equity to health

It is an anomaly that people are treated differently depending on whether they are in a private or voluntarily owned nursing home (where both their physical needs and financial needs will be assessed and met only if required) or in an NHS ward or nursing home (where they will receive free treatment and care

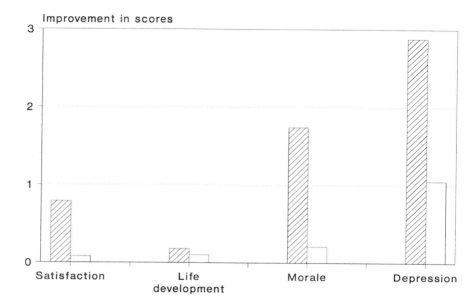

Figure 8.6 Home care (shaded) was better than hospital care (unshaded) for all measures.

without a financial assessment). The anomaly centres around the fact that there is no logical or consistent way of defining that a disabled person really needs health care rather than social care. Realizing this, the government has left it to local health authorities and social services departments to reach agreement between themselves. This means, of course, that there are 150 different definitions in the UK of who can receive long term health care. This is illustrated in Figure 8.7.

The disability characteristics of people in local authority residential homes, geriatric wards and private nursing homes were studied [281]. There were differences in the average scores for people treated in different places, with more severely disabled people in the geriatric wards and NHS nursing homes than in the private nursing homes and local authority residential homes. However, there was a considerable overlap in the degree of severity of the groups as a whole. The research workers stated that 'It is obvious from our comparisons ... in residential and hospital care that the same needs are being met'. In other words, the system does not provide equity of financial support for people with the same medical needs.

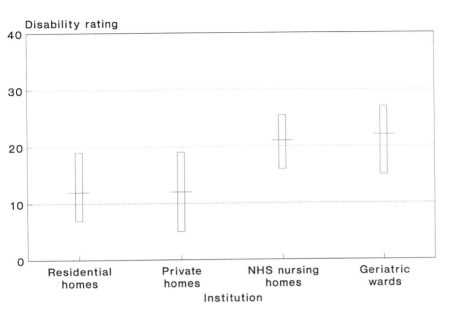

Figure 8.7 There is an overlap in disability between all of the long term providers. The horizontal line represents the mid point. (Reproduced with permission from [281].)

I have already mentioned that it does not ensure good quality care in the long term hospitals, or a reasonable way to secure sufficient funds for all elderly people who require continuous care. Several health authorities, on detecting these anomalies, have withdrawn from long term hospital care, defining the need for health care as being only short or medium term. This is obviously nonsense. A few others are developing NHS nursing homes, and a few are working on home based long term care, but not to the exclusion of residential options. Most are increasingly relying on the private sector, while trying not to think about what a need for health care really means [282].

It is self evident that the long term workhouse based hospital ward must disappear. Research findings are not important for making that decision. Health authorities are seeking cost effective, high quality alternatives. The simplest initial approach for most will be to purchase places in voluntary and private sector nursing homes.

I have concerns in this case about the lack of effectiveness of statutory controls on quality. If, as the work of Bowling *et al.* [279] suggests, there is no guarantee that a better physical environment results in a better outcome, some steps must be taken to ensure standards are met. Only the overview provided by an interested and closely involved geriatrician is likely to maintain the necessary quality of care in such small units when they have to take more people with a higher degree of dependency than they do now.

The home based approach seems to hold out much promise for the future and carefully controlled experiments need to be repeated in health authorities. Work on extra care beds in sheltered housing is progressing, but these individuals are likely to be less dependent than the population normally seen in long term beds. It is worrying that the monitoring of such developments, so far, is largely descriptive.

Adding health to life

Many long term care management proposals suffer from a lack of regular review of the people in them. This is especially common for small, scattered units and seems likely to become a bigger problem as home based care is developed. People in long term care need to remain in touch with the rest of the health and social care services. Some health authorities have withdrawn some community services from elderly people in private nursing homes. To me, this seems inexcusable.

PEOPLE CENTRED CARE OR REAL CHOICE FOR PATIENTS

When 250 people aged 75 and over, living at home in Cardiff, were asked under what circumstances they would consider going into some form of institutional care, two-thirds could not think of a situation where they might consider it. When asked if they would reconsider their decision if they were incontinent and unable to get out of bed, half still claimed that they would not. Virtually everyone questioned said that they had somebody who would be available to help them, and that this person or persons would look after them.

The main worries older people have about institutions are about the possibility of having to stay for a long time [283]. Elderly people believe that admission, to geriatric units in particular, leads to them being 'labelled'. They wish to avoid this by being admitted, if necessary, to medical or surgical wards in general hospitals. The most common disadvantage of geriatric care noted by prospective clients was the presence of other, disabled or disturbed elderly people, difficult to avoid in an inpatient service. Elderly people felt that, although private and local council run residential homes also implied a considerable loss of independence, they preferred them to geriatric units.

Studies have shown that some carers believe their elderly relatives admitted to health service institutions for long term care are well cared for. Others seem to suffer considerable guilt [284]. One reason for this must be the lack of support available to carers of dependent elderly people who are inpatients. This appears to be because no one thinks it is necessary, forgetting that visiting relatives in hospital is stressful for both the patient and the visitor. For elderly relatives it can also be extremely costly. What support is available has had a tendency to be stereotyped and limited, both in quality and quantity. It may be that home based long term care will provide the answer.

RESOURCE-EFFECTIVE CARE OR GOOD STEWARDSHIP

The costs of different types of long term care in the UK have been studied by a number of researchers. Donaldson and Bond [285] have looked at the costs of NHS based nursing homes and compared them with the costs of long term hospital wards. Figure 8.8 shows the results for adjusted figures comparing the three nursing homes they studied with local ward facilities.

The NHS nursing homes have similar costs per patient per week to the hospital wards when new. The costs of the Darlington project [280] and hospital

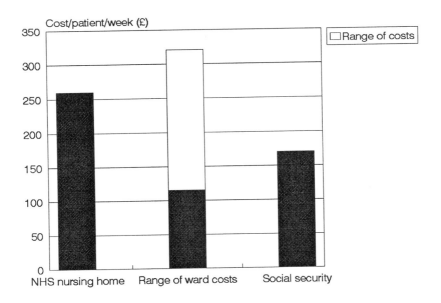

Figure 8.8 NHS nursing homes cost about the same as care in a new long term geriatric ward. (Reproduced with permission from [285].)

group are shown in Figure 8.9. The group treated at home had an average cost to the services much below that of the hospital treated group. Fascinatingly, and this may be the most crucial finding of this important, if flawed, study, the costs to the family and other carers were lower for the home managed group. Also, the families of those cared for at home were happier with the care than those whose relatives were in long stay wards.

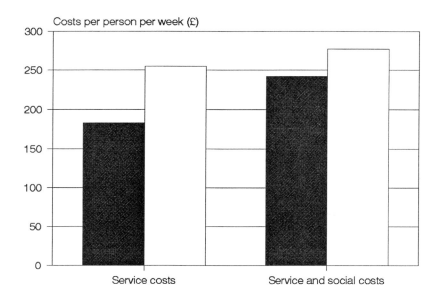

Figure 8.9 Home care costs (shaded) were lower than hospital costs (unshaded), even for families. Reproduced from [280].

Overall it appears that home care for long term care is the best option, but the research work is not sufficiently robust as yet. Careful oversight by specialists of private nursing homes may prove the best intermediate option. The presence of a consultant on the management committee is likely to be more effective than the existing system where homes are monitored by the health authorities or the Social Services Inspectorate. Such changes would provide 'homely' environments for dependent people needing long term care. It would make the units increasingly smaller, ultimately allowing people to stay in their own homes with care being provided on a domiciliary basis.

COMMUNITY HOSPITALS FOR LONG TERM CARE

The moves outlined above have the benefit of relieving the health service of having to pay hotel costs. It also means that service providers can obtain assistance from a variety of organizations, whether independent, social services or health service. This in turn allows one to get round the problem of deciding whether a patient has health or social services needs, for in the home the health services can be provided free, whereas social services can be paid for separately. A number of health authorities have been developing general practitioner run hospitals as part of their local services. Such hospitals, it seems to me, are very similar to the NHS nursing home concept if used for long term care and are therefore useful as an interim arrangement. Home care or an arrangement with a small homely unit is more likely to be acceptable to disabled people, and, according to the criteria set out above, more likely to provide increased health gain.

9

Effects of changes: patients and carers

Reducing dependence on hospitals will increase the amount of treatment and care given to people in their own homes. This will obviously increase the involvement that family members will have in caring for patients. The good news is that this will have the effect of making a closer relationship between families and the service providers. This is often misunderstood, for the evidence is that families caring for dependent people are overburdened by that care. However, a central point of this overburdening is that the service providers are not involved at all. The greatest problem for most carers is their isolation from the service providers. My belief is, that if the service providers initiate new home based services, using resources saved from hospital care, and for less dependent groups than is now the practice the whole service can only improve. The important development from the carer's point of view is whether the relationships will be more or less fulfilling at one extreme, more or less physically and emotionally overwhelming on the other. Family members and their response to any reduction in hospital care are certainly crucial to the successful development of home and community care.

It has been assumed that families will be reluctant to take on these changes in relationship and the probable increase in responsibilities that this will entail. The examples cited for this reluctance usually assume a number of things. First, that the groups of patients who will be mainly involved will be those with chronic illness, either mental or physical, and who will therefore be hard work physically and mentally for the person caring for them. The group needing care is usually assumed to be elderly or chronically mentally ill and their care burdensome. The second assumption is that for these and any other groups, hospital care is less of a burden than home or community care. The third assumption is that the provision of home and community back up services in future will remain much as they are at present. I will examine in more detail the first two assertions and the changes to home and community services which will be needed to make the new ideas work.

CARERS FOR NON-CHRONIC ILLNESS

The majority of patients with chronic illness, whether mental illness, learning disability, elderly disabled people, the elderly mentally ill or young physically disabled people are presently looked after at home by relatives [286]. The changes envisaged in this book may be expected to increase the proportion to a small extent. The information we have about carers suggests that this cannot increase greatly without a lot more practical help for families and also a change in the attitude that communities have towards families assisting with sick or disabled relatives. Such changes in the way that society works are slow and their direction is unsure. The assumptions about probable changes in the reliance on hospitals made in this book do not depend critically on piling more workload onto families caring for heavily dependent people. It is possible that the move from hospital care to community based care envisaged here may occur without any increase in the proportion of people who are caring for chronically ill or disabled people in their own homes. Part of the intention of this book is to suggest the alternatives for caring for such people, without recourse to any structure that would be thought of as a hospital.

There is good evidence that people caring for the chronically ill are not, themselves, being cared for reasonably [287]. Having said that, there are a large number of myths about the needs and attitudes of families and other people who care for mentally or physically disabled people. Carers, mainly family members, provide more than two-thirds of all care in the community. They provide care for dependent people usually elderly, physically disabled or mentally disabled. Without this population of carers we would not be able to support all those people who require some form of help with their daily living.

The *General Household Survey* of 1990, a survey which reflects the situation in all of England and Wales, questioned people caring for the sick, disabled and elderly [286] in order to find out who they cared for, their age and sex and the amount of time spent caring. Some of the findings were unexpected and at variance with the existing literature [288, 289] and the general beliefs about carers that one hears voiced in the media. It was useful for quashing some of the more important myths.

For instance, the data on carers were compared with similar data from 1985. It was found that there was little change in the proportion of those who were caring for someone else during that period. In 1985, 14% of people over the age of 16 were caring for dependent people in the community. In 1990, the figure was 15%. Contrary to the commonly held idea that a much greater proportion of women care for relatives than men, the proportion of men and women carers was 13% and 17%, respectively. Similar proportions of men and women look after someone in their own home but women are more likely to care for someone outside their own home. Women slightly more frequently took the main responsibility for caring, but there was little difference between the two surveys or between the sexes in the proportion of people who were caring for others for

20 hours or more per week. The proportion of males and females who care is similar, but because many carers are elderly and more women survive into old age than men, about six out of 10 carers overall are women. Figure 9.1 shows the number of people in the study [286] who were carers by age and sex groupings.

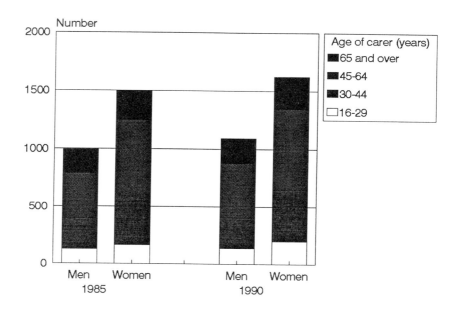

Figure 9.1 The number of carers of dependent people in 1985 and 1990 in a representative sample of the population of England and Wales [286].

Carers were most commonly in the 45–64 year age group. Of those under 45, single people were more likely to be carers. Almost a quarter of all carers spend 20 hours or more per week caring. Women tend to spend slightly longer in their caring role. In a quarter of cases the carer and the person being cared for were unrelated. About two-thirds of the carers looked after people with a physical problem, a quarter looked after someone with a mental disability, the remainder looked after someone with both mental and physical problems. Those people not living with their carers were more likely to receive care from the formal services than those living with carers.

It is to be expected that the population of carers will be focused on more and more as implementation of the NHS and Community Care Act gets underway. The Act and its implications are discussed below. As its title suggests it emphasizes the importance of people being cared for within the community wherever reasonable. Previous work has put little emphasis on the needs of physically incapacitated dependent people, the needs of men caring for dependent relatives and the contribution that statutory services are already making.

CARERS OF CHILDREN

An important group, for whom hospital care has, quietly, become increasingly irrelevant is children. The view seems to have become accepted that children, apart from the most extremely ill for very short periods, do not belong in hospital. This is an interesting group, because the carers of children have to contend with different attitudes from service providers to, for instance, those caring for chronically ill people. Carers of chronically disabled adults and elderly people have the impression that they are invisible and their contribution is not appreciated [290]. In contrast, those looking after children tend to be blamed for any difficulties that service providers meet with. Parents are said to be overprotective or overanxious, transferring their problems to the child and making inappropriate use of expensive services [291].

When parents are given specific tasks to help with the health care of their children, however, they make an important and sensible contribution [292]. The move away from inpatient care has been welcomed by parents, who often take a complex part in the care of their children, including parenteral antibiotic therapy [293], the prevention of severe asthmatic attacks [294] and the reduction of hospital visits in a number of other ways [295]. It has been shown, at one extreme, that giving more information about asthma to parents reduces the mortality from the disease [296]. The presence of parents in hospital reduces the hospital stay [297]. Parents can also carry out many of the routine caring tasks in hospital with great benefit to the child [298]. Parents, faced with children being increasingly cared for at home rather than in hospital, welcome the move and provide valuable additional help in providing care.

CARERS AND DAY SURGERY

It has been previously mentioned that surgery will be given mainly as day care in future. This is partly owing to a change in emphasis, because of changes in techniques, allowing less invasive approaches and therefore shorter recovery times. There has not been a great deal of discussion of the load that this will impose on family members, despite the fact that the Royal College of Surgeons guidelines specify that patients should not be left alone during the 2 days following a day case operation [299].

The rate of admission of patients to hospital overnight after day surgery is very low: fewer than one in 100 of those operated on [300]. It seems unlikely that a great deal of difficulty is caused to family members. One study from Australia suggested that about one patient in 700 of those given day surgery needed to be admitted overnight to hospital for social reasons, presumably owing to the inability of the family to cope [301].

Patients certainly seemed as highly satisfied with day surgery as with inpatient surgery [302] when asked afterwards. It seems unlikely that such satisfaction would be forthcoming if relatives had not been happy with the approach, though there does appear to be a gap in the research literature on this point.

CARERS AND ACUTE GENERAL MEDICINE

The remaining major group of patients, those treated in acute medical specialties, including those in acute geriatric departments is being discharged earlier, but remains an important segment of those using inpatient care. These are the groups that some of the recent hospital at home schemes have been targeting. The pressure on families from the reduced length of stay has not been pinpointed by researchers as a problem for carers.

Having said this, about one in 10 elderly patients already feels that he or she has been discharged from inpatient hospital care earlier than should have been the case [303]. This does not seem to have altered over the past 5 years or so, during a time when lengths of stay in hospital have shortened dramatically. Carers do not seem to be especially concerned about patients being discharged too early [304]. Their concerns seem mainly to revolve around poor communication and nurses' attitudes while their relative is an inpatient, and problems with the dependent patient at home. These can increase to the point where life becomes unbearable without any help from any of the services.

HOSPITAL, LESS OF A BURDEN FOR CARERS THAN HOME CARE?

There is a widespread belief that having a relative in an institution, whether hospital or nursing home, is less of a burden on families than home care. This appears to be largely the result of a feeling that the amount of work done on a hospital or nursing home ward must be impossible for untrained people. This ignores a number of differences between hospital and home care that are often greatly underestimated by professionals and the public at large.

The professional approach to the care of patients in hospital involves finding out what is wrong with patients, treating them and sending them home. Other things are secondary. Most patients and their families have a different set of priorities. For patients the priority is to be symptomless, and to be able to cope with their normal occupation and the needs of their family and friends. It is enlightening to question relatives. Husbands and wives are often very resistant to any proposal to let their spouse be cared for in hospital.

Other relatives, particularly those who have been very involved in the patient's care before admission to an institution, find that they attempt to continue to care for them when they are inpatients and this causes a great deal of stress [305]. Problems revolve around financial concerns, guilt about the decision to admit the patient to care, feelings of loss of control and a lack of self confidence in solving problems for the relative admitted. Other problems are caused by lack of support from other members of the family and friends who may blame the main carer for allowing the patient to be admitted. All of these feelings of guilt are exacerbated if a chronically ill patient expresses a desire to return home but the relative finds the thought of caring for them at home is too much. Sometimes the sense of guilt causes close relatives to distance themselves gradually from the patient [306].

This appears to be much less of a problem if services are brought into the home to assist with curing and caring. In addition, a number of studies have shown the extreme difficulty that relatives find with visiting patients in hospital. The mechanics of getting to the hospital can be extremely complex, especially for poor and elderly people. Once at hospital there seems to be nothing to do and it is difficult simply to sit by the patient, often in an embarrassed silence because of the relative's lack of knowledge of the life of the patient in the institution.

Relatives who were providing long term care to elderly people at home felt much more positive about the work than those caring for patients who had been entered into hospital care. In particular, guilt at the admission of disabled people to long term care often leads relatives to be very aggressive about the care of the dependent family member. Relatives under considerable anxiety and depression from caring for an elderly patient at home often do not seem to improve when he or she goes into an institution [307].

A large number of intervention studies have been undertaken in these areas, most of which were poorly organized and controlled [308]. Guidelines for good research in the area have been drawn up in detail [309]. It is to be hoped that new findings will help to clarify how best to help relatives caring for dependent people. Since the advent of the Community Care Act, social services departments have been developing considerable expertise. The health service has been slow to join them in learning these lessons.

NEW APPROACHES TO BACK UP FACILITIES AT HOME

Over the last 10 years there has been considerable interest in developing new ways of working with families to help them care for patients with long term disease. There have been attempts to try to develop the abilities of the family to cope. This is preferable to removing the patient or grafting in service providers who will take over for a time, then move out again. Some good examples now exist for the care of families where one of the members has schizophrenia.

This is one of the most difficult problems for families to face. New methods of family management aimed at reducing the relapse rates for patients and also maintaining the quality of life for other family members and carers are being increasingly tried [310]. Such an approach is essential if community based mental health services are to progress [311].

Many questions are raised when trying to develop a treatment service which can help the whole family. Because of this it is difficult to integrate with intervention into a full clinical psychiatric inpatient service. There have been few randomized controlled trials on the use of such family therapy and the numbers in those there have been are very small, but the approach is promising.

This is not to say that providing therapy for the whole family has no difficulties. Sometimes relatives deny the presence of mental illness in the patient, particularly when newly diagnosed. In other cases, the relative's distress is translated into anger towards the professionals involved. Newly diagnosed patients with schizophrenia are therefore a particularly difficult group to help because of the pressure that the diagnosis itself imposes on the family. Many families do not accept the necessity for family intervention. They may have a very mechanistic view of the disease and expect the service to cure the patient of their symptoms.

It has been suggested that a number of elements are necessary to make family therapy work. The first of these is that the family must be seen as being part of an informal partnership so that families and individuals feel they are involved in making decisions about what should be done. In addition, there is a need to educate the professionals about the needs of the families. In particular to give accurate information about schizophrenia and what it implies. Lastly, any interventions that are suggested by the professionals must fit in with the known structure of the family and its own interests and needs.

It has been suggested that the central issue in the treatment of people with schizophrenia is that families with high levels of 'expressed emotion' are at risk and should be a priority for family intervention. Certainly patients in families with such characteristics do tend to relapse more frequently than families with low levels. It is also known that this family therapy can reduce the high levels of expressed emotion [311].

An important reason for the breakdown of such therapeutic approaches is a lack of trained staff. A crucial function of any family therapy unit is therefore the training and development of new people to do the work. The emphasis in the work is on helping the family to develop its own expertise so that they can better deal with crises and find solutions for their own unique problems, rather than prescribing a set answer to predicaments [312].

Family members, partners in community services

When people living at home are asked what they will do if they become ill, most state that members of their family will be available to assist [313]. There are two aspects to the home care of dependent people by their families: the degree of dependency of that person and the ability of the carer to cope in physical, mental and social terms. Previous work has concentrated on the latter.

Data from some studies [314] have explored the interrelationship between the dependency of people and the contribution made to their care by relatives, friends and the statutory services. Some survey groups and methods in this field have inadvertently led to an underemphasis on the contribution service providers now make to the home care of dependent people [315]. It seems likely that biases have misled planners about the care available to different groups.

In two general practices in South Wales, 1300 patients over 70 years of age were chosen from typical urban and rural settings [315]. The need these people had for care was defined by the normal activities which they were unable to do. If a high percentage of people are unable to perform an activity, such as going shopping, this denotes a less severe degree or disability than where a low proportion of people are unable to do an activity, such as getting out of a chair. The analysis used this direct approach to dependency in order to simplify the way the needs of dependent people are described. This also reasonably clearly describes the pressure such needs put on the family and services. The tasks for which the person was dependent on others were not an exhaustive list of things that people can be dependent for. They were chosen to represent the degree of severity.

When the elderly people had been asked about the things they could not do, their dependency on others, they were also asked who helped them with those tasks. Figure 9.2 shows the number of people in the study who were dependent on others for a range of tasks from shopping to getting out of a chair. The figures for the percentage of people unable to perform each task have been placed in order. The activities chosen had to be important. In other words, if the task was not done it would mean that that person would almost certainly need someone else to do it for them or, failing that, would suffer as a consequence.

The tasks form a gradation in severity, with the task which suggests that the person is most severely dependent, being unable to get out of a chair, at the right, the least, not able to go shopping, at the left of the line.

This increasing severity fits with another simple classification of dependency, the interval method [316]. Using this method, those said to have 'critical interval dependency', need care at any time at irregular intervals. They correspond in Figure 9.2 to those who would be unable to get out of a chair or walk indoors. These people therefore depend on others for other important tasks, most importantly going to the toilet.

Those less severely affected are said to have 'short interval dependency'. They require assistance at least once a day. This describes those who are unable to cook, go outside, bath or climb stairs. The most essential help that such people require is for obtaining food, keeping warm and keeping clean. Those with less severe dependency are described as having 'long interval dependency'. Such people are unable to perform actions which need to be completed

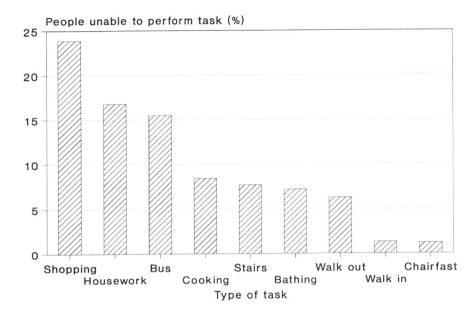

Figure 9.2 Percentage of people over 70 unable to perform certain tasks. Reproduced from [315].

at least once a week, such as doing housework and shopping. The scale can be used for any group of people, whether physically disabled, mentally ill or learning disabled, though for the mentally ill further information on dangerous or disruptive behaviour is usually included.

Figures 9.3 and 9.4 show the dependency data compared with the age of the subject for men and women. There is a clear gradation with age. Older people are more dependent on other people than younger people for all of the activities. The figures show the extent of this with different age groups and emphasize the high prevalence of dependency in the oldest.

The proportion of women who are dependent is greater than men in virtually all of the groups illustrated. There is little difference in the order of the tasks between men and women except for cooking, where women score better than men at all ages. The proportion of men who are severely (critical interval) dependent in the final two categories is considerably smaller than the proportion of women. In terms of the actual number of people this represents in the country as a whole the difference between the sexes is even more extreme, as far more elderly women reach the older age groups than men.

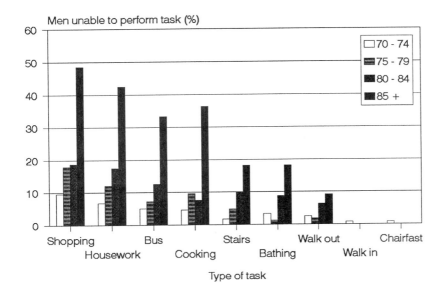

Figure 9.3 Proportion of men aged 70 and over unable to perform certain tasks. Reproduced from [315].

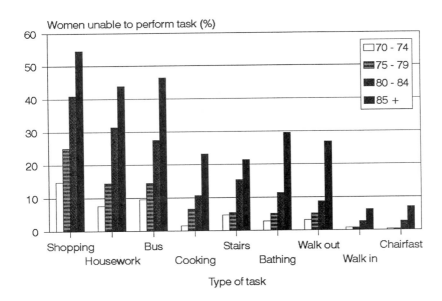

Figure 9.4 Proportion of women aged 70 and over unable to perform certain tasks. Reproduced from [315].

Figure 9.5 shows the percentage of people who were dependent and who were assisted by different people, family members or service providers. A single unpaid person, usually a relative, was the commonest type of carer, making up the majority of those who cared for this group of frail people. These individuals, as shown in the detailed right hand figure, are most commonly daughters, followed by the elderly person's spouse and then a range of others.

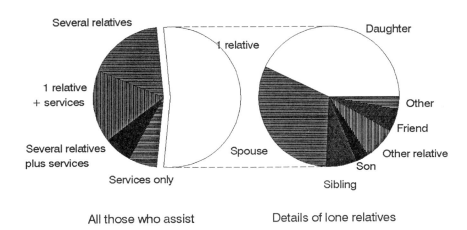

Figure 9.5 Most of those who care for dependent people are lone relatives. Reproduced from [315].

For about a fifth of dependent elderly people, more than one unpaid person shared with helping. A further fifth of the elderly people were assisted by one unpaid person with the help of an official service, for example the health or social services. For about a tenth, more than one member of the family or a friend shared with a service provider and for a tenth official services alone provided assistance.

Figures 9.6 and 9.7 show the details of the degree of dependency for men and women by whether assistance was provided by relatives, services or a combination of relatives and services. There are important differences between those with mild or severe forms of dependency. In the most severe categories no one was cared for by the official services alone. However, the proportion of people cared for by a single person, who was virtually always a relative, decreased markedly as dependency increased. The groups with several relatives together

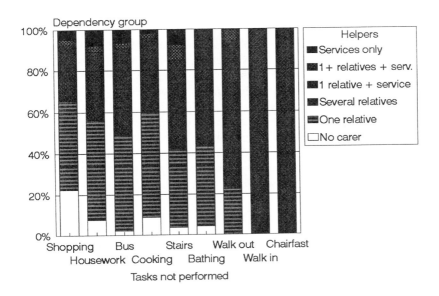

Figure 9.6 Proportion of dependent men and who assists them. Reproduced from [315].

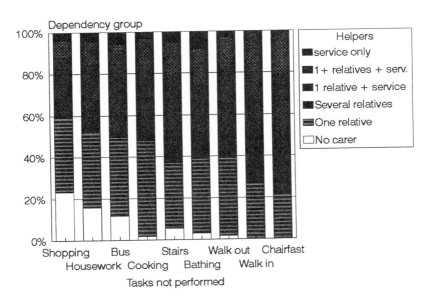

Figure 9.7 Proportion of dependent women and who assists them. Reproduced from [315].

and relatives in combination with services increased as severity increased. In other words there was a marked trend for more people to become involved as the elderly person's dependency increased.

These analyses show how complicated is the relationship between a dependent person living at home and those caring for him or her. In these figures one person, usually a daughter or spouse, makes a major contribution to caring. However, it also shows that the official statutory services increasingly help with caring for highly dependent people.

Many previous studies have concentrated on the pressure on carers, paying relatively little attention to the severity of the dependency of the elderly person or relating the one to the other. There has also been a tendency to oversimplify the carer's role by concentrating on the main carer and ignoring other subsidiary helpers. This tendency has continued in a number of recent studies on those caring for dependent people. In some studies, data have been obtained solely from men and women already getting services, including those newly discharged from hospital, people in day centres and carers groups [317, 318]. One suspects that the main reason for this is that the data collection is simplified because such people can easily be identified and questioned. Such groups of people will be biased by families who are either well informed or caring for the most severely dependent elderly people, where service intervention has been sought or is so vital that the family would otherwise break down if help were not given.

Other surveys [319–321] have been made on the needs of those who care for dependent people, highlighting the costs to the family of performing such tasks and the degree of stress experienced by family members. This approach is valuable from the carer's perspective but does not always lead to an obvious conclusion about whether official services are already available and how new ideas can be developed to relieve the situation. When carers are asked what they need they often lack information about what is available and therefore simply suggest more of the services they already receive.

The complexity of the relationship between dependency and those who care for the dependent person has also led to an underestimate of the contribution of service providers. The presence of services at the household of elderly dependent people suggests that these services can be further developed to alleviate the problems of those caring for elderly people at home. However, they must be made aware of their own potential for developing better customized services.

RESPITE CARE

Social and health service professionals tend to see the primary purpose of a relief break as being to provide a time for carers when they do not have to think about the needs of their dependent relative [322], but this is an oversimplification of the possibilities. These may be to provide a holiday or rehabilitation for dependent patients themselves, who may be conscious that they are a burden. It may be to cope in an emergency situation and to prepare or assess dependent people for the inevitability of long stay care. Breaks may be occasional and irregular or on a rotational basis where the elderly person spends a set number of weeks in care and the intervening period at home.

A popular form of respite care is the use of day centres or day hospitals. There is a strong feeling [323] that hospitals should not be used for relief care but should be kept for rehabilitation. This is to avoid an important function of respite care, as a time when rehabilitation can be carried out. There is evidence that about a third of patients attending day hospital are there largely for 'social' purposes, usually to give families some time away from their dependent relative. It should be said that day hospitals, with the requirement for patients to be ready for the ambulance early in the morning and for the carer to be ready for the patient to return home in the evening, both times being within a wide range and varying from occasion to occasion, can often cause more problems for a family carer than the relief implied by the visit to the hospital.

There have been complaints in the past that the day care provided by voluntary agencies for elderly people is less stimulating than that of local authorities [324, 325]. Some local authorities have learned to encourage the voluntary sector to produce small day clubs which are professionally supported and highly appreciated [326]. Some people have suggested providing day hospital and day care on the same site, with the advantage that a psychogeriatrician may be available to support the elderly mentally infirm patients [17]. This type of organization is rare, but as hospital assessment and inpatient care diminishes it is likely to become the norm.

A complete break is possible at a residential home, hospital or assisted lodgings. Local authority old people's homes have been increasingly making this available and there are now more short stay than long stay admissions in some areas, including my own. The development of the Community Care Act has increased this provision further in some places as it is government policy that local authorities should obtain most of their services from the independent sector. The relatives of some dependent people are able to get away on a holiday by paying for a nurse to live in. This does not often seem to be available in the public sector and usually seems to depend on personal contact between a relative and a suitable nurse. For very dependent people it seems like a sensible approach for the future.

Demand for respite care

A number of studies have shown that a third of the people looking after a dependent person would have liked support from the social or health services, but had not received respite care [17]. Many did not know how to go about obtaining such care and a number did not know that such a service existed. Places available are often not taken up, partly because of a reluctance by services to advertise what is available in case they become swamped [327].

A number of researchers have suggested that information about relief breaks is very haphazard. Elderly people and their carers who were aware of the existence of such breaks were likely to apply for them. There is some suspicion among the general public that elderly people receiving relief breaks do so because they are in some way particularly favoured, especially those that go into hospital. Those who use social services short stay care are poorer than those who do not and older than average. They also have more severe disabilities in general [328]. Those going to short stay holiday homes were less dependent than those who went into social services short stay provision.

A striking finding from surveys of respite care is that very few old people who received such care were being looked after by their husband or wife. This appeared to be due to a fear of an adverse affect on the dependent spouse and the fear of loneliness in the spouse carer. They seemed to see the looking after each other as part of their marital role and suggested that relief care would undermine their self respect [329]. Children appeared to be much more willing to take up assistance. Some type of respite service which is acceptable to people caring for their dependent spouse obviously needs to be developed.

Attitudes to respite care

In general, relatives are appreciative of care wherever it is provided, in hospital, homes or assisted lodgings [330]. A major problem appears to relate to rotating care, that is short periods in a unit giving respite and short periods at home. Some researchers have found that relatives who most benefited from rotating care actually wanted the person they were caring for permanently admitted to residential care but put up with rotating care as second best. A number of relatives appeared to improve in terms of their mental health when the person they were caring for was permanently admitted to care or died.

Research workers have been critical of the way that elderly people are prepared for respite care [287]. They showed that some families needed more advance notice that a place was available and more information about what had happened to their dependent relative while they were away. For instance, some dependent frail people had suffered falls while in respite care but there was often no report of this, or it was mentioned only in passing. There was some concern among relatives about the flexibility of the care, for instance some was not available at weekends.

The people in charge of some private residential homes felt that their regimes were not really suitable for short stay care. However, elderly people in such homes appreciated the stay and valued, in particular, the food and sometimes the company. They rarely felt that it was a holiday. Opportunities for reassessing their needs or providing rehabilitation were not available in private care. Some respite care residents felt that the homes that they went to were depressing, particularly the state of other long stay residents.

It has been suggested that respite admission to hospital for social reasons or a holiday admission is often associated with acute illness and quite a high death rate among elderly people. One study goes so far as to suggest that such admissions should be discouraged because of the danger of cross-infection [331]. Residents who have experienced short stay care in both private households and residential homes generally preferred the former, in lodging schemes for instance, though this did vary greatly, depending on the quality of the residential home [332]. Many carers are themselves elderly or disabled. There must be a considerable need for assistance for both the dependent person and his or her carer while remaining together, either in the family home or on an accompanied holiday.

Breakthroughs in respite care

Families and other carers are not homogeneous groups but are highly diverse in terms of their age, income, housing, education, area they live in and their access to health and social services. In planning different types of respite care the needs and preferences of those who are not getting help as well as those who are receiving it need to be taken into account. There is evidence, for instance, that those caring for elderly people in rural areas have different needs from those in urban areas [333]. Respite care may meet the needs of some people but would be more fitting if it was widely and more regularly available, especially at awkward times or at short notice. Instead it is seen, both by those providing it and those receiving it, as some sort of prize in the face of extreme adversity.

Perhaps most extraordinarily there appears to be no work on what mentally or physically disabled people themselves prefer as respite care. We do not know if they have preferences about whether respite care should come from voluntary sector organizations, health services or local authorities, whether they feel that they are receiving charity or whether they would regard making a payment as more acceptable.

Some of the research into the needs of carers is now out of date. Changes in the ownership of houses, reductions in the home help service and in public transport and the wider ownership of telephones and cars will have changed the needs and problems faced by elderly people and their carers significantly over the last 10 years. Many social services departments are now reluctant to provide housekeeping services, concentrating their efforts on people who need help with personal care, such as washing and getting to the toilet. In this way, many people employed by the social services are carrying out tasks previously done by nurses while abandoning their traditional home help and meals services.

More flexibility is certainly needed. Disabled people have different needs in the summer than in the winter. Carers may have different needs depending on whether schools are on holiday or not. A most imaginative but simple scheme has been set up in The Netherlands. This happens to be in a nursing home, but the approach is equally applicable to small grouped homes or even in the home of an elderly couple. The service was set up so that the elderly dependent people ran a crèche for the children of people who were looking after them. This freed the parents to work, looking after the old people.

Workplace programmes for employed carers

The families of dependent people have considerable difficulties staying in a job. If the development of community care is to be a central point of the way that health services evolve, these problems must be taken into account and ameliorated. Relatively little has been done in the UK to assist carers outside the provision of crèches for mothers of young children. In the USA, however, quite a lot of work has been done on relieving the burdens caused by care giving and trying to work.

In a series of studies of employees, one-fifth to one-third have been found to be caring at home for dependent, usually elderly, people. The competing demands of work and caring for a dependent relative can cause considerable difficulties for many care givers [334]. A fifth of people who are in this position reported conflicts with their work: they sometimes have to work fewer hours, rearrange their schedules or take time off without pay. These problems were related to the degree of disability of the person that they had to supervise [335]. Other problems included lateness, absenteeism, unscheduled absences from work and excessive use of the telephone. It has been reported that promotion opportunities, training and job changes were inhibited by having to look after a dependent relative [336].

Family carers have suggested ways in which their problems could be eased. A large firm in California asked its workforce how it could be assisted. The employees stated that flexible working and allowing time off for family illness would be most useful. In addition, one-third of the people caring for dependent relatives suggested that a programme of information on the needs of disabled people given by the company would be useful [337].

Recent surveys have shown that employers in the USA are becoming more aware of the difficulties faced by members of their workforce who are caring for dependent people [338]. Some companies have policy leaflets and programmes about child care that can be adapted to apply to that of other dependent relatives. Over two-thirds of firms in a recent survey in the USA offer unpaid leave of absence for people to care for parents or children [339]. Almost half of the firms offered flexible hours and a third were willing to give part time work during the period that this was needed. This has improved considerably over time with over twice the number of firms offering flexible work schedules in order to care for elderly people in 1990 compared with 1989 [340].

Federal legislation is proposed in the USA which would require employers with 50 or more employees to provide up to 12 weeks' unpaid leave for family or medical reasons while maintaining the employee's benefits and guarantee of a job. A number of states in the USA require employers to provide unpaid leave for this purpose. It is estimated that this costs employers $35 million annually for days off to care for seriously ill parents and $142 million annually for days off to care for ill spouses. A number of insurance packages aimed specifically at helping those caring for dependent family members have been set up. Almost a quarter of employees of medium and large firms were eligible for assistance [341].

A number of very large firms, notably the IBM Corporation have information and referral programmes where guidance in locating community services such as nursing homes, meals and medical care are provided for employees who need them. The information services are usually provided free of charge. Some companies have also set up employee assistance programmes which give counselling and information on the needs of dependent, particularly elderly, family members. A few companies have sponsored self help groups.

The Striderite Corporation in 1990, in what has become a famous move, opened an intergenerational day care centre for employees. This accommodates young children and elderly people. It has opportunities for children and the elderly people to work and play together in various ways, as well as providing separate areas for different activities. If there are spaces free they can be taken up by the local community residents, either children or elderly people.

The International Ladies Garment Workers Union has organized a service where women who have recently retired from work have been given the chance to train to provide respite services for union members, giving temporary relief from care giving responsibilities. Other firms have helped their employees by donating money to local community services. These innovative far-seeing approaches are obviously in the interests of the private companies which are supporting them as well as being of inestimable value to the employees themselves and to the local health and social services.

Private sector employers in the UK have been virtually unaware of the needs of employees who are carers [342]. There is a feeling that the large health and social government run organizations overwhelm local initiatives, whether from industry or the growth of large scale voluntary work in the community. There has for many years been a feeling in the UK that voluntary services in health and social work are temporary phenomena, while the service proves itself, when the statutory services can take over. Where they are better organized, voluntary service providers usually depend heavily on money from social services departments to keep going. One firm that is an exception is Marks & Spencer plc, which is launching an elder care policy for staff, a trust fund to assist those retiring and work site services, such as information, fairs and employee counsellors.

10

Effects of changes: quality assurance

CARE AT HOME: UNIQUE QUALITY PROBLEMS

In some ways the quality of services given appears to be better for non-centralized than hospital based care. This is especially the case for the amount of information and explanation given to patients, a central concern of both patients and their families. Despite this, any move towards home care will need, as part of the service, strong action to ensure that quality is maintained. There are unique characteristics of care at home or care in small, localized, homely units that make the monitoring process different from what is needed in an inpatient unit.

Firstly, patients looked after in this way who are elderly, very disabled or mentally disabled may be more vulnerable to individual fraud and abuse in a small unit where there are few other patients present. It may be argued that relatives or friends are more likely to be present and would be more alert for such misuse of trust than other members of the same team in large units. There are situations when patients do not have carers present where the care given at home or in small units is essentially invisible to everyday scrutiny by other people. However, the problems which have come to light in the past appear to stem from small closed communities which remain stable in terms of their staffing and patients over long periods, when odd or even dangerous traditional practices can develop. Classically the problem areas have been long term nursing homes for elderly disabled people [343]. This is despite the fact that they are, and have been for many years, more closely regulated than any other service in the UK [344] and the USA [345].

I have mentioned that, in practice, patients treated in their own homes or small local units have a greater degree of knowledge of what is happening to them and what they can expect. Luckily progress in giving the general public and patients more information generally appears to be gaining ground. If this continues, patients and their families will be much better able to judge whether the treatment and care that they receive is of a reasonable standard.

Quality begins with the values held by the organization providing the care. This approach is being explicitly required of the NHS Trusts and Social Services Departments for the first time as a result of the NHS and Community Care Act [346]. The existence of such written values does not, of course, guarantee that these will be followed, but it is a start. Purchasers of services, whether general practitioner fundholders or health authorities are putting explicit standards into their contracts with providers of services. These are slowly but increasingly being developed as a result of asking the local population, especially people who have recently been patients, what standards they would like to receive.

The traditional method used for looking at the quality of the UK health service has been to examine past actions in detail where they were imperfect in some way, usually as a result of a complaint or series of complaints from a patient. The assumption was that people who gave poor treatment or care in the past are likely to be continuing to do so. Any suggestions for improvement or disciplinary action should concentrate on this area of the service.

It will be obvious that the difficulty with this approach is that the worst may already have happened. The enquiry can only concentrate on trying to stop it happening again. Legislation relating to health is often brought about as the result of particularly horrifying scandals which receive a great deal of media attention. Such scandals, because of their extreme nature, are often unique and result in complex changes being made to the way that health care is organized to no great purpose.

REVIEWS OF WORK TO IMPROVE QUALITY

Peer review is a method, set up originally by medical consultants, to try to identify bad practice before it causes harm. This involves setting a defined standard of care and collecting data about when it fell short of what was expected. The treatment of blood pressure, for instance, has been judged against a number of criteria, one of which was whether three abnormal readings had been collected before treatment was started [347]. The emphasis in this case was on the large number of cases where this triple reading had not been carried out, in order to underline the large proportion of cases where good practice is lacking.

This approach, requiring the collection of large quantities of data, has been simplified and is now universally required in the UK and USA, where it is known as medical audit. A better description of what is required would be a formal review of procedures. Quality in this approach is often largely seen as a double negative finding. If none, or only a small proportion, of the things identified as undesirable are present the treatment or care must therefore have been not bad. This means that there is a possibility for hiding incompetence as the information is gathered. The people providing the service may spend time concentrating on the particular audit processes which can be monitored, giving less time to other, less tangible, and therefore less measurable, parts of the work.

Setting standards: the use of guidelines

The development of clinical guidelines is an approach to improving the quality of care that has been used in the USA for some years and has recently increased in popularity in the UK. It may concentrate on the positive side of setting out best practice in some detail. It relies on experts to help set up the guidelines, sometimes with advice from patients or patient organizations. Here too there is often a list of things which should not happen.

The best guidelines have the advantage of cutting across different specialty boundaries, giving advice on which parts of the service can be given by general practitioners and which need specialist care. It is assumed that adherence to the guidelines will improve the standard of care and therefore the well-being of patients. In the UK, the Royal Colleges have been very active in setting up such approaches.

This technique seems to fit in with the development of community based care, for the guidelines include directions about what can and cannot be attempted in hospital or in the community, given the amount of expertise available locally. The best guidelines are therefore locally set up, or at least local modifications of national guidelines. There is a problem here for comparing the way that services are carried out in different places, but this appears to be inevitable if guidelines are to include, as the best ones do, details of the management of the service, and do not simply restrict themselves to the nuts and bolts of therapy.

Guidelines have been produced for a very wide range of diseases. There are analyses of the effectiveness of different methods of diagnosis, treatment and investigation ranging from such things as effective care in pregnancy and childbirth [348] to the long term care of elderly people. Clinical guidelines or protocols have been used in the USA and Canada for some time to try to control the behaviour of the medical profession and, in particular, the cost of health care [349]. The experience of the American Medical Association and American College of Physicians in this field is therefore considerable. The greatest problem appears to be to get the guidelines adopted in practice [350]. Doctors have to be exposed to the same message in different forms. Those devised by senior doctors are often felt by their junior colleagues to be unrealistic in practice or likely to fail [351].

The system of purchasing and providing in the UK lends itself to the use of guidelines, for purchasers can specify that they wish particular diagnostic therapeutic and other procedures to be followed. This has not previously been a dominant theme in the purchasing of services [352]. Therefore, it is premature to say whether putting a guideline into a contract is a more persuasive method of getting professionals to follow the guidelines than the peer pressure of their colleagues.

There are some other problems. Guidelines are often over-cautious in their recommendations and can result in patients being over-treated; their treatment can be extremely costly. An example [353] was found in the recommendations of the British Pacing and Electro Physiology Group which suggested that the use of complex pacing was necessary in heart block and suggested a particular piece of equipment which was extremely sophisticated. The authors of the paper felt that using such equipment on a predominantly elderly population would be disadvantageous both in terms of the needs for follow-up of those elderly people and the increased cost.

A great number of studies have tried to put together and then test guidelines for the use of laboratory investigations. A large review has suggested that such guidelines are variable in the impact they have [354]. Some guidelines suggest the negative approach alluded to above, that certain things should never happen. An example of this has been in the use of neuroleptic drugs in patients with learning disabilities [355]. There is no evidence that such medicines are of any use for such people and they have considerable risks. Guidelines which suggest that such treatment should be used only in exceptional circumstances are reasonably easy to follow up.

The Americans are now much less sanguine than the British about the use of guidelines, possibly because they have had longer experience with them. A number of professional organizations in the USA have developed a uniform style towards guidelines and it is widely felt that a national standard for most of the decisions made by doctors and other health professionals will develop here. The driving force in the USA has been to reduce costs and to avoid the legal difficulties that physicians there face if they do not follow standard practice. These pressures are not as important in the UK. It remains to be seen if purchasing can be an effective alternative.

One observer [356] suggests strongly that guidelines which control what is done to patients are enough, whether the patients get better or not. The best was done, so no more can be asked. The author also says that guidelines that state certain activities should not be undertaken are more likely to be supported by scientific data than those that suggest activities that should be. He also suggests that most of the choices made in such sets of guidelines are set by policy rather than by scientific data.

Guidelines may be especially effective when they specify which grades of staff should undertake particular types of work. This is easier to organize and to monitor than the details of diagnostic or therapeutic activity. A good example is cited by Moote [357]. He mentions that guidelines for pain control are plentifully available and most are carried out by nurses, once the regime has been set up by the medical staff. The author makes a strong plea for the wider use of guidelines, underlining that pain control is not difficult, it is simply often badly done when left for each case to be managed as if the rules for pain killing were being reinvented each time, often poorly.

There is a particular problem when more than one set of guidelines is developed for a disease. An example of this is seen in asthma [358], where guidelines have been altering over recent years but are still not uniform in different places. This is less of a problem in the UK where, with less available, it is reasonably easy to pinpoint which organization should be controlling the guidelines. The Royal Colleges have done a great deal of work in this area and have tried to make it their own. This has not motivated doctors to comply with the guidelines [359].

In some areas, guidelines have been greatly assisted by the development of meta-analyses to back up the scientific data which is necessary for ground work in the area. An example is in cardiac rehabilitation [360], where matched analyses have shown that rehabilitation reduces cardiac deaths and sudden deaths. Those with a low risk of further heart attacks are shown to benefit best by modification of their risk factors, particularly smoking.

PROBLEMS OF QUALITY INHERENT IN HOSPITAL CARE

There are a number of problems for hospitals attempting to improve the quality of their care, which appear to be inherent in their make up. In the past, quality issues have been ignored as irrelevant to the central needs of patients: to be diagnosed, treated and rehabilitated safely. Much has been sacrificed in terms of the patient's short term comfort and well-being to allow the experts (doctors, nurses and therapists) easy access and freedom to act, in the belief that this freedom is essential for the professionals to use their skill to the utmost. This, in turn, was believed to be the best thing for the patients in terms of their survival and fitness long term.

Two years before my father died, inoperable cancer had been diagnosed during a 3 week stay in hospital. The stay almost killed him. The food was unpalatable, the bed uncomfortable, the heat of the ward unbearable, the noise at night a constant drain as it kept him awake. The procedures necessary to perform the simplest acts, such as going to the toilet and shaving, needed to be negotiated carefully, both with other people and the physical layout of the ward. He had nothing but praise for the staff, it was simply an awful environment for care.

Once taken home he received his favourite food, overcooked or undercooked according to his preference, consisting of a large proportion of home grown produce. He looked out on a view he had chosen years before, an environment he knew intimately. Friends and acquaintances visited, who would not have done so had he remained in hospital because of visiting hours and transport problems. Few of them would have relished sitting embarrassed for the required half hour, no more no less, beside his hospital bed.

These things, which appear to be virtually impossible to reverse within a hospital environment, are important for the general well-being of patients, but can also have a direct effect on the speed at which they get better. The problems are not isolated. As an example, inadequate intake of food is a considerable problem for patients in hospital. A recent study of 500 patients admitted to a teaching hospital in Dundee [361] showed that two-fifths of the patients being admitted were undernourished and a third were overweight. When patients were reassessed on leaving hospital it was found that, on average, patients had lost about one-twentieth of their weight during that time with the greatest weight loss in those who were originally undernourished.

The patients came from a number of specialties and had a wide variety of different diagnoses. Such problems are not new. Evidence obtained from other studies which showed malnutrition in inpatients in general medical [362] and general surgical [363] patients have been known for many years. It is known that such poor nutrition is not only bad for the general morale of patients but increases their morbidity [364] and, not surprisingly, their length of stay in hospital [365].

There is no excuse for such nutritional negligence in hospital, but it is a symptom of the approach which suggests that technical methods of diagnosis and disease treatment are all important. I suggest that this approach is inherent in the hospital system, not simply part of poor management. Training in the needs of patients for adequate nutrition, or, indeed any other socio-medical, rather than bio-medical, need is virtually non-existent. They are certainly not seen as an important part of the care of patients, either on humanitarian grounds or as a means of hastening patients' recovery [366]. It is obvious that such approaches can be modified, indeed are reversed to a degree in some wards in some hospitals. The easiest way to alter this for all patients in all wards is to stop using hospitals in this way.

INFORMATION FOR QUALITY IN PRIMARY HEALTH CARE

Because of neglect it is difficult to find a list of randomized controlled trials which have been carried out in primary health care and which could form the basis of measures of quality. There is no standard method of obtaining this information. Silagy [367] examined a computer based method of searching the literature and discovered that no journal had a system that allowed identification of all the randomized controlled trials it published in primary care. When the journals were searched by hand instead of using the computer database it was found that it had missed up to a third of trials. Given this difficulty in finding out about publications Silagy suggests the need for a centrally based register of randomized controlled trials so that primary care can develop, based on good and easily obtained information. Another author [368] has pointed out that general practice research is a minority activity and suggests that in future health authorities should set up a strategy for research and development aimed at general practice and be encouraged to take part in research in the future.

General practitioners have been asked which clinical problems and types of measure they thought would best reflect their ability and how satisfactory care had been for their patients in general practice. A number of different areas which could best be used for such work were suggested by 98 general practitioners [369]. The three clinical conditions which general practitioners thought were good measures of their own ability were asthma, diabetes and high blood pressure. They suggested that success should be measured by the level of function of the patients, that is their lack of disability. They went on to suggest that a good measure would be the ability of general practitioners to prevent these diseases from getting worse. An alternative measure of quality would be the number of complications caused by the treatment or the doctor's intervention. Another measure should be the extent to which patients understood their condition and their resulting quality of life. The importance attached to these differences varied depending on the disease in question. Figure 10.1 shows the details. Patient preferences can be quite complex, varying from disease to disease, but understanding of the disease process remains a priority for all of the diseases examined.

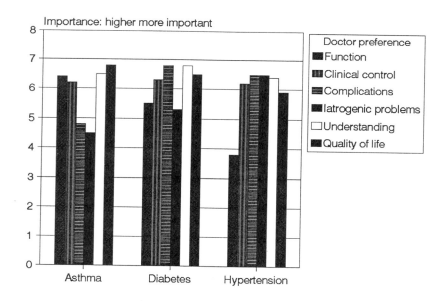

Figure 10.1 Patients see different things as important, depending on the disease in question. (Reproduced with permission from [369].)

QUALITY FOR HOME BASED SERVICES

In a study of home based care versus hospital care for patients with severe mental illness [370], it was decided that important factors would be the likelihood of these long term care patients dropping out of treatment and being lost to the service. Another approach, used in maternity services, was to ask the patients what they thought were important aspects of the service [371].

Most of the women regarded the continuity of midwifery care, such as in the domino system, where the midwife delivers the baby in hospital and then continues to care for her at home, as very important. A very high proportion of the women considered a home like environment in the delivery suite to be important and suggested how this might be done. They particularly disliked the 'clinical' atmosphere of delivery units which appeared to be more like operating theatres than units in which an essentially normal process was to be carried out.

Patients require more information

If facilities for treating people are to be smaller and more distributed and if general practitioners will be able to choose between these facilities, it will be necessary for patients to have more information about the quality of the medical care they can expect. In the USA during the 1980s, it was believed that price competition between different providers would cause the services to improve. As prices became closer together it was believed that providers would compete in terms of the quality of the product that they produced. The purchaser–provider split was to some extent set up in the UK with this as an aim.

A knowledgeable general public served by a fundholding general practitioner, in the UK, should be able to choose their general practitioner and via him or her those aspects of a service which are important to them. These might include its accessibility, effectiveness or quality. The purchaser–provider split and the internal market has, or will shortly, develop much more information on the costs and quality of services provided by different trusts. This is certainly not comprehensive at present but the pressure to produce and ultimately to publish such data will be difficult to resist.

Patients will be unlikely to choose service givers who cannot give information about the quality and cost of the service they have available. There is therefore an opportunity for individuals to obtain and make use of data about quality in different hospitals or community units. It is likely that organizations will develop which will help patients to make sense of the data. Most patients will need help to decide what quality measures are important and how to compare different trusts.

The most important measure of quality for patients is the outcome; their chances of survival and getting better. Almost as important is the process that they have to go through during the care and patients tend to concentrate their criticism on this area [372]. Patients in the UK have a tendency to regard the central part of their care (the quality of their diagnosis and treatment, their chances of survival and being fit at the end of the process) as taken as read. This may be because they feel that they do not have the expertise to judge between different professionals or hospitals once they have made a decision about which one to ask for help. This is not to say that patients do not, in theory, pick and choose beforehand. Simply that once the decision is made the technical part of the visit is taken as read.

Some people have tried to help the general public by giving them standard sets of data about the ability of different professionals or hospitals. Traditionally there have been three groups of measures relating to quality of care [373]. The first relates to the structure or input side of the care, the facilities available, the degree of training of the personnel, the ratios of staff to patients and so on. The second relates to the processes carried out, for example the administration of the service, as suggested by waiting lists and difficulties getting to see the professionals. The last aspect can be split into two. First, the outputs of the service: the number of clinics or patients seen. Second, the outcomes for the patients: the proportion who survive and the proportion who feel better and for what length of time. This last measure may include the likelihood of a patient getting back to work or leading a normal life.

Much of this work has been carried out in the USA, largely because patients there who are moderately well off have had more choice of who to go to than patients in the UK. They can simply pick or choose any facility in the knowledge that their insurance system, or their own bank balance, will meet the costs. There is therefore a body of knowledge about the preferences that patients make, given a reasonably open choice. British and American patients will, of course, have different views on what aspects of their care are important, set partly by their expectations. The approach is described as a method of giving patients information about quality rather than emphasizing the actual results. Some of the measures are universally applicable.

Sisk and colleagues [374] chose 10 basic measures to show the quality of care given by both physicians and hospitals:

- hospital mortality
- adverse events (e.g. infection from hospital)
- disciplinary action against doctors
- sanctions from peer review
- malpractice suits
- doctors' performance treating specific diseases
- number of services available
- external evaluations (e.g. neonatal care)
- specialization of doctors
- patients' assessment of their care.

As I suggested above, some of these measures would be irrelevant to patients in the UK, emphasizing the problems of trying to draw up a list which will cover different societies. Some are obviously very important, but others, such as sanctions as a result of an official peer review, do not exist in the UK. Others, such as malpractice suits, are rare in the UK.

A similar list relevant to UK practice can be suggested. Many of the measures are not routinely collected at present in the UK, especially the routine and objective measurement of a physician's performance in treating a specific disease or set of diseases. Interestingly the mechanism for doing this (medical audit) now exists in the UK. Indeed, it is a mandatory activity, but the results are not published outside the local group of clinicians involved and are certainly not for public scrutiny.

It seems likely that in future the auditing process will become a broader activity, involving teams of nurses, doctors, therapists and social workers, instead of the doctor based, rather solitary, variable quality discipline that it is at present. There will be increasing pressure from purchasers to obtain more objective and comparable data on audit activities which will be published. In addition, good provider trusts will be keen, as part of their increasingly important marketing activities, to make their abilities available to purchasers and, ultimately, the general public. Clinical audit will be a central facet of this information, together with the methods that they have developed for dealing with backsliders.

Letting people know about quality

In the USA, the federal government provides assistance to hospitals in the Medicare and Medicaid programme and also obtains from those hospitals information on the quality of their care. Simply making this publicly available would cause a great deal of controversy and would tend to discriminate against some hospitals which might, for instance, take on more severe or particularly unusual cases than others.

The first thing that is required for making information about hospital care or community care available is that the problems of interpreting the data should be explained. This has been rephrased in some circles as meaning that some kind of ultimate measure must be available, which will encompass all the possible factors which might improve or reduce the performance of a unit. This is not possible. Fairly raw scores with a written interpretation are possible and will be as far as most data can be stretched.

The press in the UK are not particularly good at interpretation. In general, they tend to take the views of experts at face value without a great deal of critical analysis. Some merely look for scandals which will provide useful headlines. At best the media will obtain the views of two experts, usually giving widely divergent views, and will provide little synthesis of the resulting argument. This may have succeeded in making the general public wary of the views of any expert. There are a tiny number of exceptions to this, usually on radio, which prove that an interesting but objective view can be given. However, such approaches do not seem to have a powerful effect on reading or viewing figures.

Picking up data from the media or relying on experts providing the service is not very useful for helping people to make decisions about the type of health care they want. Nor does it help them choose between different possibilities, including the central point of this book, how and when to choose between hospital and community care. Traditionally, general practitioners have carried out the task, often with little consultation with their patients. To be fair, the majority of patients have been happy to accept the general practitioner's decision, or at least, have not voiced their opposition.

Purchasers and consumer groups with experts on their staff, who are able to explain the important issues to the public, would be better placed than individuals to analyse the quality of care information and to persuade providers to improve the care they give. This is certainly one of the functions of the purchasers in the new purchaser and provider climate in the UK, but it has not been given priority compared with trying to balance the books. Few consumer groups have really taken on the process of analysing the quality of care given by different hospitals. A few Community Health Councils have asked their local populations about the services provided locally. However, these questions have tended to be quite superficial and often badly worded. The development and delivery of questionnaires about satisfaction with health services is a task for people with some experience in the area.

To compare information about the quality of different hospitals or hospitals versus community care, the data must be simple and accessible to people. Individuals who are feeling ill, or who have been informed that they have a serious illness, are not capable of analysing large amounts of complex data about where they should go. In addition, people need skills and some social support to ask physicians about the quality of care in different places.

Curiously, although the quality of care is possible to measure in a number of ways, little research work has looked at whether making the information available actually influences what people choose. This appears to be because the information is so rarely given to patients, even as a research project. In the UK, few patients know that it is now possible for them to choose, without restraint, their general practitioner or via their general practitioner which specialist they can see.

In the UK, the fundholding general practitioners make contracts with certain consultants for specialist care. There is some concern that this might in fact reduce patient choice. General practitioners tend to refer cases to consultants they know and have worked with in the past. It is important therefore, that general practitioners should be aware of the importance of their choice and that this point should be put strongly to them, both by patients, before they need care, and by consumer groups. On the other hand, it is not in everyone's interest for consumers to move constantly between different hospitals or physicians, as measures of quality are produced from unstable data, showing different service providers at number one in the medical hit parade.

Assessing quality depends on the participation of the majority of health care professionals. It is therefore important that they should not become defensive and attempt to undermine the system of assessment. If bad physicians are seen to be getting good assessment and good physicians bad assessment, the system will quickly be brought into ill repute.

The UK government has begun a process of making available to the public league tables of hospitals according to certain criteria [375]. The criteria used in the first set of tables in 1994 were based on waiting times for different procedures in different parts of the hospital system:

- patients seen in outpatients (percentage in 30 minutes)
- accident and emergency assessment (percentage in 5 minutes)
- operations cancelled (readmitted within months of second appointment)
- day case surgery (percentage of hernia, knee examinations, cataracts, sterilization)
- waiting times (percentage admitted for surgery in 3 months).

The publication of these tables led to considerable controversy from the Labour party opposition on the grounds that they were not related to patient outcomes. Some doctors said the tables did not give a full picture. It is interesting to speculate on the outcry that would follow if a fully comprehensive set of validated health outcomes were produced!

The government did not, as is essential, give a detailed commentary on the strengths and weaknesses of the indicators and an explanation of how they could be used by the public. In particular, they did not make a judgment on the right length of the different waiting lists. Local conditions could also cause the data to be unavoidably biased, and this was not explained. Nevertheless, the data are an interesting start and it was probably right to publish them with detailed discussion coming later. For interest, the figures for day treatment of cataract surgery, a subject mentioned earlier as being especially well suited to day work, are shown in Figure 10.2. There is a huge variation in the proportion of patients treated in this way.

THE PROFESSIONAL POWER BASE IN HOSPITAL

There are obstacles to removing the hospital dominance of the health care system and developing secondary community based care, primary care and care in the home. The most complex of these come from the definition of professional roles [376]. A few professional boundaries have been nibbled away. For instance, some nurses have taken on some of the roles of doctors, as nurse practitioners, and some auxiliary nurses have been allowed to perform more complex work than they have before. These changes have been minor compared with those needed for the degree of change that appears to be inevitable.

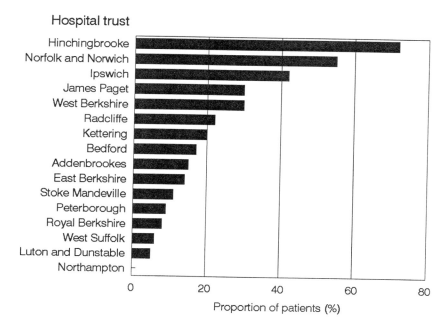

Figure 10.2 Patients receiving day care for cataract surgery in the Anglia and Oxford regions. Reproduced from [375].

The UK health service is starting at the top with the gradual re-merger of district and family health services, recognizing the importance of the overlap between primary and secondary care. On the provider side, a number of hospitals have developed community based services, realizing that they need to have a powerful say in community based care. This is to ensure a rapid and efficient throughput of patients and to control their waiting lists for admission and the type of admission that they take. Yet, for the people actually seeing patients, there are still problems with differences in professional rivalry. Also, in the UK, there is an enormous division between health and social care. Health is largely free at the point of delivery and social care is becoming more expensive. This is at a time when the objective difference between the patients or clients seen by either is extremely difficult to define. Social care in particular is becoming steadily more interventionist, more concerned with personal care and the relief of disability, while medical care appears to be moving towards rapid intervention and away from long term care.

The district general hospital and the more generalist functions of the teaching hospitals will have to learn to behave flexibly and, to a degree, avariciously. Failing this, they will find it difficult to exist over the coming decade. Primary care and community based secondary specialists will gradually widen the margin between what has been traditional inpatient and community based care. The move must surely be, if not on cost grounds, on the grounds of convenience and patient preference, towards the community.

The more complex functions which district general hospitals carry out are increasingly likely to be overtaken by specialist units which may be quite large, regionally based organizations or may be a loose federation of super-specialist units kept in touch with one another by a modern communications system. If we wish the changes outlined here to come about without a major upheaval in the professions, as they resist them, we need to look ahead at how professionals can best be prepared. Retraining will obviously be essential to the change. The UK has never been particularly good at such an approach, preferring to give early retirement rather than to try to teach people who are brilliant in one field how to be brilliant in another. This is a waste that we cannot afford.

THE PRESSURES WILL BE IRRESISTIBLE

Health issues are already important news stories in the UK and throughout the developed world. This means that any information publicly available about the quality of care will rapidly be transmitted by the media. It seems likely that the public will demand high quality care much more than they do at present. This process may be accelerated by the availability of self diagnostic and self treatment services using the telephone or personal computers.

The process of computer diagnosis is developing slowly but in fairly narrow areas at present. It is quite conceivable that within the next decade private medical companies will be available to give advice over the telephone and shortly after that the whole process may become automated. This will mean, at the least, that people will be able to get a second opinion for most of their primary care, even if they do not have access to a full diagnostic treatment service.

Richard Turner [377] has presented a futuristic but quite feasible possible approach with the description of 'mediphones' in a shopping complex. These are able to refer to a patient's previous record while taking a relevant history about the symptoms presented, sample his or her breath from the mouthpiece of the telephone, do an ECG and examine his or her internal organs using ultrasound. It will also test eyesight and, by linkage to a local chemist, prescribe treatment.

The most unlikely part of this scenario is that the various computer data bases, including that of the tax office, had been linked up! The citizens of the UK have long been extremely reluctant to allow any such linkage, and presumably it will take many years before they give way on this point. It does seem, however, quite likely that private companies may set up smaller versions of such a diagnostic service. There has been a preview of such changes, with pregnancy diagnosis and cholesterol measuring kits now being available from chemists, despite some professional opposition.

Doctors, who may be resistant to travelling to patients rather than having the patients travel to a central point to see their doctor, will not need to move. Indeed, if such a system is set up much larger numbers of people will be able to be cared for in their own homes and fewer professionals will be needed for diagnosis and treatment. The few giving direct hands on treatment will remain with those supervised caring services, especially nursing in the community.

Pressures for quality from general practitioners

The development of fundholding general practitioners acting as purchasers of services for their patients is leading to an important change that I have not mentioned. The task of fundholding general practitioners is to manage the budget for certain categories of patient, at present those who require routine inpatient treatment and certain community services.

There will be financial pressure on fundholding practitioners to manage at home any patients on the margin of being admitted to hospital. This power is being given to fundholding general practitioners, but, spurred on by the development of fundholding, some district health authorities are finding it sensible to work in collaboration with non-fundholding general practitioners in order to assess the needs of their population and to set up contracts with local providers. This will help to speed up changes in the way that services are provided.

It will therefore be in the interests of general practitioners to provide, from their own practice, as many services as possible. This is likely to hasten the change in emphasis from a hospital orientated, inpatient and secondary care led service to a primary care led service, with secondary care acting as support to primary care. It seems likely that the hospital services will act as a support to the main specialist, secondary services, which will be based, not in hospital, but in the community.

Fundholders are increasing in number but district health authorities still purchase the emergency services and services for non-fundholding general practitioners. It is still the job of the health authorities to oversee the quality of most of the care given by hospitals. In Hackney [378], the general practitioners have developed ways of getting the views of other general practitioners and hopefully those of their patients back to the health authority. In this way, even general practitioners who are not fundholders can ask for particular types of service which may be lacking from the hospitals.

In Hackney, this works through a general practitioners forum. All the general practitioners in the area are invited to monthly meetings which are held at different surgeries in turn to encourage everyone's involvement. Only two practices in the area have chosen to become fundholders so far, possibly because of this ability to intervene with the health authority. Advisory groups were set up to advise the health authority in the early stages, but as with many such groups they lapsed for lack of support. In 1992, the Family Health Services Authority agreed to fund an administrator and seven adviser posts of one session, half a day, each to carry out this work. The general practitioners have met monthly and have made links with specialties which have an important part of their work in the community. The work they have done includes attending joint planning meetings, working on clinical guidelines, audit and education activities. As a result of this the practitioners have a clear view of the way that service planning at the health authority meshes in with the actual service provision.

This is seen as a way of setting up a commissioning partnership between general practitioners and health authorities which might offer some of the benefits but none of the risks of fundholding. Most general practitioners in Hackney feel that the forum expresses their views and that it does have an effect on the way the health authority presents its plans.

A more significant change in the way that general practitioners' work is being piloted in Bromsgrove in Birmingham where four general practices have been given a budget of £13.2 million to buy all the health services for 40 000 people [379]. The budget has been handed over by the North Worcestershire Health Authority to fund all of the needs of Bromsgrove's residents. This includes emergency services, ambulance services and maternity services. The belief is that general practitioners who see patients every day are more sensitive to patient needs and can therefore use their budgets more flexibly. The four practices had already been fundholding practices, buying routine hospital treatment for their patients. The project has been run by a committee of four general practitioners, one from each practice, and the Director of Public Health for the area together with the Chief Executive of the Health Authority. A team of researchers is monitoring the progress of the pilot scheme.

CHANGES WILL HAVE TO BE MANAGED

The focus of this book is on the decay and diminishing importance of hospitals, with many of their functions being taken over by community based secondary and primary care, the former centred on specialists, the latter on general practitioners. Many of the remaining hospital functions are likely either to become centralized, as for pathology services and some intensive care, such as transplant services, or divided up in small local units, such as day surgery.

This scenario may seem too doctor orientated for many readers. They may point to the development of multi-disciplinary teams, the extension of nursing skills and practice, the increasing importance of social work in purchasing and providing community care services, or the growth of the powers of a management class, as evidence that people other than doctors will be central to the provision of services in contact with patients. While I believe that specialist consultants in hospitals or in the community will be much more restricted in their freedom to manage their own patients in future, I think it is unlikely that doctors as a group will lose a great deal of the power that they wield at present. The only move that may block the central position of doctors is if they deliberately abdicate the responsibility by refusing to take part in the changes.

Groups of general practitioners may prefer to give their power to a manager to make decisions on the best services to buy and get on with being providers of primary care to their patients. It is, after all, what they expected when they took up the job. Consultants may refuse to come out of hospital as the main part of their contract, so that others take up the oversight of the secondary acute care. There are many waiting for such opportunities. Nurse practitioners, pharmacists, chiropodists, therapists, social workers, specialist technicians would all gladly take on more responsibility if it also allowed them access to a small proportion of a consultant's power and salary.

Some decisions have already been made which, in the UK, will result in consultants losing some of their standing with increases in their numbers and reductions in their junior staff. These are proposals agreed under the Calman Committee report, which suggested a reduction in the number of junior staff working in hospital and an increase in the number of specialist consultants [380]. Despite all this it seems unlikely that doctors will give away the opportunity to stay in charge of what remains to them.

The change towards community care is to a large extent inevitable but, as with all changes, the effect of the changes on those working in the service can be reduced considerably by some forethought. It is very fashionable at the moment to talk of 'managing change' but there is a school of thought which suggests that achieving change is what managers are for and that unless there is change managers are superfluous.

Management is not about the preservation of the status quo, it is about maintaining the highest rate of change that the organization and the people within it can stand.

Sir John Harvey Jones

It has been suggested that the ability of an organization to respond to change is a measure of its health [381]. The health service in the UK in the last 10 years has been asked to change more completely and more rapidly than it has since it was formed in 1948 and the rate of change continues to accelerate. The difference between the recent changes and previous upheavals in the way that the system has been run, is that change now appears to be built into the structure. In particular, the division of the health service into purchasers and providers means that purchasers have the ultimate sanction of removing money from the provider if a service does not meet the expectations of that purchaser. This will put pressure on providers to adapt to the demands of the purchasers. Purchasers will inevitably be faced with reductions in the amount of money available and will therefore induce those providing services to be more efficient, closing down older schemes in order to start new ones with the money.

Many of the recent changes in the health service have emphasized the importance of managers and managing as a process. This is largely because it is believed that using professionals, particularly doctors, to lead the service results in piecemeal unplanned changes reflecting the interests of the specialists with the greatest say. It is felt that the interests of the local consultants would bias the service in their direction, rather than following the needs of the population. In particular the specialists, because they are specialists, tend to re-emphasize the importance of secondary and tertiary care within hospitals. It appears that the only way to bring about a reduction of the power of hospitals is to reduce the influence of consultants within those hospitals. A better way of bringing this about for the benefit of the consultants, would be for them to realize that their ability to survive may depend on their giving up hospital status.

There are a number of forces which are very powerful within the health service. In particular the coherence of different professional and specialty groups, alliances made between people who are working in specific fields. There are, for instance, groups of researchers or people who are involved in teaching and training and more natural groups, such as people of a certain age group who may meet socially. These may restrict the amount of change that is possible [382].

It has been suggested that humans are not rational. They will not be reasonable about a plan to reduce or take away their jobs, whether or not the boss believes it to be rational or if government policy dictates it to be rational. A number of policies in the past which have attempted to expand community and primary care or to develop services for the mentally ill, the learning and physically disabled by moving resources from the acute sector have foundered, mostly because they ignored these internal pressures. There seems to be at least some agreement that one of the most important parts of bringing in a new policy is a careful analysis of why there needs to be a change [383].

Once having decided this there is a need for a detailed breakdown of how exactly the policy is to be brought about. Analysing what needs to be done, deciding on the course of action and bringing it about seem to have to be done one after the other. In fact, the three are often interwoven and there may well have to be some compromise about the final outcome of the change [384].

Change appears easier to implement in some types of organization. It has been suggested that a rigidly hierarchical management set up cannot easily cope if changes are being brought about rapidly. In the health service at present there is a fashion for broad hierarchical structures with a relatively large number of managers at each level, but not very many levels. Nevertheless, within that structure of management the hierarchy is fairly rigid, with a large number of professional groups which are closed to people without long and complex training.

There have been suggestions that organic management structures fit in better with the type of pressures on the health service. In this sort of system, project teams are formed in response to a particular problem and are dissolved once the problem has been overcome. Membership of the team depends on expertise not position in the hierarchy [385].

The complexity of the present structure means that conflict is inevitable. In particular, the division between purchasers and providers in the health service is there to encourage conflict [386]. Plant [387] has suggested a method of looking at the way groups take to changes. He suggests (Figure 10.3) that one should look at who the winners are, who the losers are, who has the power and who has the information for bringing about change, in order to give information on groups and coalitions in an organization. Individuals respond to the threat of change with concern that they may lose their position or their job.

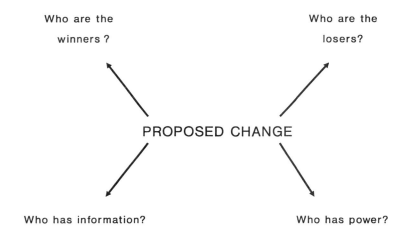

Figure 10.3 Relationships in change.

Changing the central pivot of the health service from hospitals to the community will result in a considerable number of winners and losers. The main winners will be the general practitioners who will need to run larger and more complex teams of people. They will have to develop or buy in considerable management skills. The process of moving towards fundholding has started a great many general practitioners along this path. It seems likely that the new management responsibilities given to general practitioners will allow them to continue to develop their practices into much larger organizations in the future, with educational and social work aspects for prevention and the social, caring side of the work. The time appears to be right for these changes to come about. Until now it would have seemed unlikely that general practitioners could have even approached the changes that they have already conquered.

The main losers will be the specialist consultants in so far as they will be expected to undertake a high proportion of their work outside hospital and there will be considerable changes in their present practice. There will be more of them, with fewer junior staff. They will be expected to do much of their work in the community, in ambulatory day units associated with groups of general practices or in small neighbourhood hospitals, or overseeing one or more teams of hospital-at-home groups.

The super-specialists are likely, with the development of the internal market, to cluster together in small high tech units, either regionally based with all of the super-specialists together, or with small numbers of them in different places. The groupings of super-specialists are likely to cut across traditional lines. Thus, cancer specialists will tend to cluster around radiotherapy units, with complex surgery and specialist chemotherapy given on the same site. Cardiovascular units will have as their centrepiece the necessary theatre and X-ray equipment for cardiac diagnostic work and cardiac surgery. These units will, for now, continue to develop in and around the main teaching hospitals. It is likely that the internal market will quickly show that such high powered approaches are not cost effective in the existing district general hospitals.

Identifying who has the power (Figure 10.3) at the present time is difficult. For the past 10 years the government has been willing to wield power against considerable opposition from doctors. Yet the doctors are still taking part. They have not felt that all-out conflict would be successful. The memories of the coal strike of 1984 in the UK possibly taught an important lesson.

Consultants still have their traditional power base, the Royal Colleges, but these have been relatively quiet except to claim that the service is underfunded. Within the service the purchasers, both fundholding general practitioners and the health authorities, have the money and the ability to alter the direction in which it flows very rapidly. It has been suggested, rather to the surprise of those involved with the setting up of the internal market, that up to three-quarters of the providers of services in one region are in competition with others for the services that they provide [388]. This suggests that, once they get their methods of contracting sorted out, the commissioners will be able to exert considerable influence on the way that their providers work and will be able to move resources from hospital to community care fairly easily if they wish.

The information (Figure 10.3) is not obviously in the purchaser or provider camp at present. There has been some concern that providers, who generate the information by their actions, would be resistant to allowing this to be seen by other providers or even their purchasers. This latter problem can easily be got over by simply making the information required part of the contract. Resistance to change can be reduced by the degree of confidence people have in the individual group bringing about the change, often at a very personal level. An essential part of any planning or change process is that some people within the organization will be personal friends and will therefore be able to bring about change more rapidly and with more confidence in each other than people who are not [385].

Change has been brought about in the past by employing people who have satisfactorily changed their own practice to assist with the process in other areas [389]. This has worked reasonably well, though there is a tendency for the new approach to 'slip' back to the old way of doing things if local champions cannot be found and helped.

11

Effects of changes: training

TRAINING THE HEALTH PROFESSIONS IN A COMMUNITY SETTING

It has been known for many years that large hospitals do not provide the best place for the training of their staff. Figure 11.1 shows some evidence of this from the training of nurses and sickness absence [390]. The research workers found that the nurses felt much less well orientated in the large teaching hospital than they did in the smaller peripheral hospitals and units where they did their attachments. This was despite the fact that the large hospital was increasingly familiar to them as time wore on, whereas the small units were different each time. This is a measure of the often quoted comment that smaller units are 'more friendly'.

The majority of medical graduates work in primary health care, whereas the bulk of their training is in secondary care. This is a tradition which stems from the foundation of the first teaching hospitals around the monasteries and later from the concentration of the most eminent physicians and surgeons in the voluntary hospitals, where their teaching and services to patients were free and seen as a form of philanthropy. The need to give more emphasis to primary care, as treatment is increasingly carried out in general practice, has led a few medical schools to alter radically their approach to the teaching of medicine. Some of the teaching is still given in large establishments associated with a large hospital, but most of it is carried out by primary care physicians.

The emphasis on primary care in these medical schools also carries with it a great emphasis on the rights of patients. This is parallel to the comments that patients receiving home treatment have made, that such care seems to give patients more autonomy and that professionals respect them more. In the medical schools with the new approach, a great deal of attention is paid to the preparation of students before they meet patients. Examination of the eye, for instance, is carried out first with dummy eyes, then with volunteers, then with

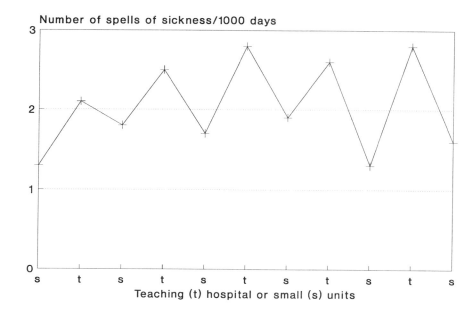

Figure 11.1 Sickness absence in nurses was greater in a large hospital than in small units. Reproduced from [390].

patients. Great care is taken that students introduce themselves and put patients at their ease. This contrasts with my own training: I was presented with a patient, whose eyes had already been dilated, and shown how to use the necessary instruments to examine the eyes on the spot. We were never introduced, largely because of the needs of the rapidly forming queue of other undergraduates waiting for a turn.

The approach to training in the new medical schools may be called the McMaster approach, after the pioneer school in Hamilton, Ontario. This appears to be a better method of training for the majority of our future professionals. Coincidentally it is also much easier to adapt the training for when hospitals are no longer the dominant force in medical practice. The emphasis on primary care puts that approach at the forefront of medicine. The careful preliminary training, before a student is allowed to have direct access to patients, allows the student to work with more confidence with patients on a one-to-one basis, which is the norm in small locally based day units or in the patient's own home.

Training for secondary care

The medical officers of North Staffordshire Infirmary in 1864 urged the use of general practitioners for teaching medical students including those who would later become specialists [391]. This proposal is still being worked on, but in the UK has not got very far. I have mentioned that medical education is being increasingly seen as having a number of important problems. For training specialists, training in medicine is seen as mainly a scientific discipline. This has two main consequences that are a problem for young specialists: the plethora of new scientific data which are constantly being produced and are, often unthinkingly, passed on to them to learn; and an unwillingness to question what they are taught. This is especially a concern in medicine where the method of working has evolved over the centuries, carrying with it a great deal of ineffective dogma, which is passed from master to apprentice. There is little time for socio-medical rather than biomedical teaching. This tends to simplify such issues as the treatment of alcohol or drug misuse and diet. As a result, doctors may fear or despise patients with these problems. They will also have some difficulty communicating information to patients, or being able to understand the complexity of patients' reactions to grief or fright.

The situation is not all bad, however. I have mentioned that some medical schools are trying new approaches and developing them over the long term [392]. It has been recognized that part of the problem comes from the selection process, where academic excellence is judged to be the first priority for entry to medicine despite the fact that much of the work undertaken by doctors is not academically taxing. Some medical schools have seen difficulties implicit in this approach and have altered their selection process so that they welcome applicants with any academic and professional background and require moderately good academic performance but not necessarily in a medical subject.

These schools pay particular attention to the personal qualities and life or work experience of the people entering their programme. Applicants are observed in a simulated tutorial and a great deal of information about the individual applying is collated before a final selection is made. As a result of this selection process many medical undergraduates have previous experience in other fields, more than half are women and the average age is greater than that for other medical schools. They also tend to favour a great deal of teaching in a primary care and community setting.

Educational methods used in hospital based medicine favour traditional inductive reasoning following the collection of a large number of facts. However, it is known that pattern recognition and the testing of hypotheses are more usually used by doctors when reaching decisions. With the decrease in the numbers of patients coming into hospital for care and lengths of stay getting shorter, the population of patients seen in hospital is getting more ill. In addition, increasing subspecialization within hospitals means that it is very difficult to get a broad view of the type of medical problems that exist in the population.

Some of the greatest problems facing medicine as a whole are ignored in the average medical course. These include, the escalating costs of health care, growing public dissatisfaction with doctors individually and the profession as a whole, the imbalance between the use of high technology medicine and primary care, inequity of access to services, wide variations in the quality and quantity of medical care, and the lack of training on how to measure whether patients have actually recovered.

There have been suggestions that there should be increasing medical education for teachers and the combination of medical and nursing teaching by a 'zone' doctor [391]. It has been suggested that clinical teaching for medical students hoping to specialize should also be done in the community [393] with teaching about the community at large and the non-medical influences on health, poverty, ethnic origin and environmental factors being emphasized.

The most important advantage that teaching from general practice has is that disease and disability can be studied in their natural context. This should make it easier for teachers and students to avoid assuming that exotic diseases are common and that diagnostic categories are clear cut and easily obtained. The latter is a particular danger in hospital when the student sees a patient who has been looked at by a number of people and has had a large number of investigations performed, so that the process of reasoning is in reverse. The patient is presented, when he or she has had a diagnosis confirmed. The student's task is then to elicit the classical signs and symptoms of that disease and to suggest treatment. This is a particular danger for students who will become specialists, for they will learn to ignore patterns which do not fit the established set.

The approach may have been useful in some, probably mythical, era when most patients were acutely ill, were diagnosed, treated and then became better or died. It is certainly in stark contrast to the present day reality, where most patients have a series of interlinking problems, many of which are untreatable. A decision has to be made about whether the available treatment will, on average, help these problems rather than hinder them. If the treatment is complex, a judgement may have to be made about whether the patient is likely to accept it.

GENERAL MEDICAL COUNCIL PROPOSALS

Stirred by these developments, the General Medical Council (GMC) in a recent report [394] recommended considerable changes in the way that medicine is taught in medical schools in the UK. The report makes the point that the main focus of medical education up to now in the 20th century has been understanding disease processes as they effect individuals, diagnosis, and management. It stresses the reawakening of the wider interest of 19th century doctors in the health of populations and the epidemic, social and environmental hazards that affect them. The GMC says that public health is to be reinstated as a priority subject in the planning of medical services.

The report describes a shift in the balance between hospital based services and those providing general practice. They point out that in future there are likely to be more overlapping skills and responsibilities. They also emphasize the importance of teamwork among professionals and the priority to be given in future to learning to train aides and relatives, who may have little or no training except for carrying out specific tasks for a single relative. This type of approach will be important so that expensive professional skills can be used to their best advantage.

The GMC report also states that there has been a drive within medical education towards an unrealistic degree of completeness. Medical graduates, on the day they graduate, have been trained in every specialty that they may later wish to enter. The GMC suggest that, as all specialties now require higher training, most of the factual learning in the undergraduate course can be brought in at a later stage. They also point out that the knowledge base of medicine changes quite profoundly over short periods of time, so that the ability to relearn and adapt is more important than absorbing today's facts.

They also suggest a reduction in the total amount of knowledge that medical students need to learn. They put emphasis on a required 'core' of learning and closer integration of the scientific part of the undergraduate curriculum and the part which has always been traditionally taught as an apprenticeship system.

These recommendations are similar to changes that have been brought about in the 'McMaster model' medical schools. Another parallel with the approaches of these new medical schools is the emphasis on project work and the requirement for students to study in some depth a small number of aspects of the work that they do. This would not be the same for all students, indeed diversity in the approaches that different students take is to be encouraged, apart from the core itself. Another principle is towards self-directed learning. Preparing the programmes necessary for such an approach requires a lot of resources in the early stages but this is thought to be compensated for later, both in terms of the flexibility of the course offered and the time that teachers need to spend on it.

Other parts of the GMC recommendations suggest the crossing of traditional departmental boundaries so that interdisciplinary collaboration in planning courses will tend to break down the barriers between traditional specialties or will at least lead to new alliances between different groups. There are particular suggestions that medical students should be brought into contact with families in the community in which, for instance, a baby is expected or which contains an elderly or disabled member. The recommendations point out that skills are more important than knowledge for good medical practice, as knowledge can alter rapidly in science and suggest the development of two new important areas of work: the idea of man in society, and the importance of public health. They suggest that there should be much more emphasis on the importance of the prevention of disability and minimizing handicap during the rehabilitation process.

The move away from hospital, outlined in this book, means that there will need to be much more emphasis on training in primary care, particularly training by and for general practitioners. It suggests that all doctors, particularly general practitioners, will have to think hard about the jobs they perform and therefore the training they will require for those jobs.

GENERAL PRACTITIONERS AND THEIR FUNCTIONS

When looking at training one needs to bear in mind what will be expected of doctors in future. General practitioners will be expected to undertake a number of different tasks at any one time [392]. The first of these is to act as a care provider for individual patients and is the traditional task of doctors. Second, with the increasing development of screening for the detection of problems before they may have developed into full blown disease, there is increasing emphasis on those who, for instance, do not seek care but who could benefit from it and who may be at risk in the future.

In the past, the belief that disease and normality are separate entities has undermined the development of this side of the general practitioner's work. The central question that doctors have asked themselves in the past has resolved itself into whether the patient is abnormal or normal. This is not a useful approach for the prevention of disease. Pickering in 1968 [395], first described the problems. A number of measurements taken from patients show a range of grades in different people without any symptoms of disease, whether low or high. He described the difficulty of interpreting, for example, blood pressure measures, for people who have no symptoms. Yet, as is shown in Figure 11.2, the higher the blood pressure the more likely people are to have complications, without any special point at which the measure suddenly becomes dramatically more dangerous. He made the point that doctors find this idea hard to deal with. They want to know whether to treat or not to treat; no in betweens. In some frustration, he suggested that doctors can count up to two; to treat or not to treat, but not beyond.

In a number of other diseases the continuum between disease and normality is, in the same way, not easily divided into normal and abnormal. Hospitals and clinics have been able to ignore the continuum because the patients who are seen in them are survivors of a selection process so that only the most severely 'abnormal' actually arrive in the hospital or clinic. First, patients have to decide to seek help, usually from their general practitioner. Then the general practitioner has to decide whether to pass them on to the hospital consultant. In some teaching hospitals the majority of patients seen will have been referred from a consultant in a non-teaching hospital. Most research work is done in teaching hospitals, by which time only really 'abnormal' patients are seen. Primary care and some casualty departments where patients arrive as a result of only one screening process (their own) see a much broader set of patients. These decisions, to see the general practitioner, to be sent to the outpatient department, to be admitted to hospital, have been graphically described by Goldberg for mental

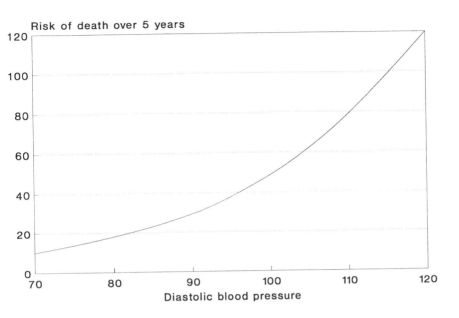

Figure 11.2 The higher the initial blood pressure the greater the risk of heart disease later.

illness, as a series of 'filters' [396], with the more seriously affected individuals moving on to the next level.

Knowledge of the difference between those seen in hospital and the general population has been described as the 'iceberg phenomenon'. The tip of the iceberg is composed of those patients who come for help to specialists. Specialists and clinicians in hospital find it natural to work on the exposed tip. Cynics might say that the patients who are allowed into the teaching hospital are more likely to be those who are unusual, rather than the most severely affected. This approach, concentrating the greatest expertise on the most ill, or those with the greatest risk of dying, is sometimes known as the high risk strategy. This identifies people who are at much higher risk than the general population. Because the risk factors that we can identify and alter are not very specific for most diseases, most of the people who actually get the disease will be in the lower risk groups. It has been suggested, for instance by Rose [397], that three-quarters of social disability related to depression may be found in people who, when tested, had a degree of depression which does not fall into the 'abnormal' range. Figure 11.3 shows how this works in a hypothetical case for the risk of suicide in patients with different degrees of depression.

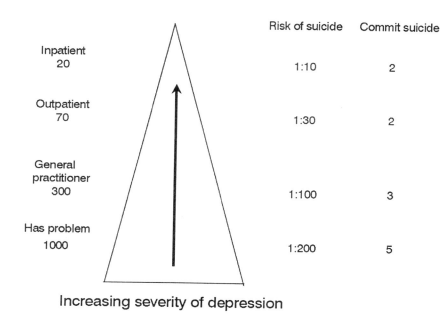

	Risk of suicide	Commit suicide
Inpatient 20	1:10	2
Outpatient 70	1:30	2
General practitioner 300	1:100	3
Has problem 1000	1:200	5

Increasing severity of depression

Figure 11.3 Risk of suicide in patients with different degrees of depression.

The figure shows that of 1000 people who have depression (which would, if seen by an expert, require help) about 300 are treated by their general practitioner, 70 are referred to the outpatient department and 20 of these are admitted to hospital. At each of these filters the more severe cases pass on. The risk of suicide is much greater in the more severe cases, but because of the greater numbers at low risk at the lower levels more people actually commit suicide in the community than those in touch with the hospital service.

The quandary is whether to concentrate on those at high risk with specialist intensive care and prevent a few suicides or to concentrate on trying to help the very large number of people with relatively mild depression, where one can potentially prevent more people committing suicide. Most health services try to do a bit of both. Although an analysis would reveal which approach is most beneficial as far as costs, the pressure to maintain a particular service may be as much due to pressure from politicians or the local population as to its effectiveness.

A similar example is found when studying alcohol intake. Groups of people who have a high prevalence of very heavy drinkers also have relatively high average alcohol intake overall [398]. Cutting the average intake of alcohol in the population will therefore also be likely to have a reducing effect in the extreme users. A further example is in the measurement of the symptoms of dementia in elderly people, where it may well be that the best means of treatment of this, presently irreversible, disease may be to work with those not 'abnormal' but showing early signs of potential problems in order to give therapies that have been shown to be of little use in the full blown disease. This approach is also most likely to be effective at giving assistance to their families and preventing the situation at home from reaching crisis point [399].

Doctors as educators

All doctors need to be educators. General practitioners, in particular, are the local experts in matters of health and illness for the whole community, the general public. The general practitioner is the one individual in regular contact with a high proportion of the local population whose position is recognized and understood by them. It may also be thought of as his or her job to act as an advocate for the community locally, taking responsibility for causes which might improve the health of the public. This has not been an important part of general practitioners' work in the past. Indeed the political nature of this approach has always been against the natural inclinations of general practitioners who are trained in person-to-person contact rather than working on behalf of groups. Public health physicians have taken up such causes in the past and are likely to continue to do so, but they are a small cadre and are involved in deciding the health needs of their population at the level of the purchaser. There remains some antipathy between the two groups.

What is needed from the primary care team, the general practitioners in particular, is the provider side of public health medicine. A good example might be work to reduce the number of girls under 16 years of age who are smoking. This has been identified as an important area for improving the health of the population by the purchasers, especially those in public health. That group might campaign, for instance, to increase the tax on cigarettes, but it is likely to be in the primary care setting that the campaign can directly reach the girls themselves. Traditionally this has been a task designated to community nurses, particularly health visitors, but they are becoming more closely involved in the day-to-day work of primary care.

General practitioners need to work closely with public health consultants, who collect the data about which diseases are common and which habits are most associated with them, and need to be particularly aware of the health of the patients who make up their community. Nevertheless, general practitioners must also take on many of the tasks common in public health to understand fully the population implications of the work that they do. To this extent general practitioners are required to act as planners or at least to be able to coordinate their own work with the plans of the wider district. As an example, campaigns to improve and help the general mental health of their patients may need to be set up with other general practitioners.

HOSPITALS AND PREVENTION

In all of this the hospital has, traditionally, played little part. People who enter hospital have been through at least two decision processes, the decision by the patient, often assisted by family or friends, to go for help and the decision by a general practitioner to refer the patient to hospital. In some specialties, especially those treating illnesses closely related to smoking or drinking, a hard line is sometimes taken in preventing a recurrence of the illness. There have been threats by cardiac surgeons that they will not treat patients unless they give up smoking. Such approaches are quite effective at persuading individuals to stop, but do not have a great deal of effect on the disease in general.

TRAINING IN A HOME BASED SYSTEM

It is much easier to understand the relationship between organic, psychological and social aspects of disease in patients when they are at home. The relative importance of these different parts of disease is more obvious and a way of sorting them out is easier to find when the surroundings are taken into account. Patients can be followed from their home through any hospital care they may require and back again, which makes much more sense than the present day 'snapshot' of the patient in hospital.

Graduates from schools which are pioneering these approaches, especially McMaster in Hamilton, Ontario and Newcastle in Australia have been found to have better analytical communication skills than graduates from schools with the more usual training programme. Improved communication skills have been shown to improve accuracy of diagnosis, the skill which conventional schools put at the top of their achievements. The advantages of training medical students in general practice would reflect in another way. The general practitioners would be less isolated and would, by the nature of the teaching, be required to work closely with epidemiologists and pharmacologists for the higher level of skills in those areas. It would put the medical students in much closer contact with the views of the general public and local community organizations, an area which is completely absent in most medical undergraduate training. There have been some suggestions that the 'world should be turned upside down' over the past few years [400], but very few actual changes have occurred until recently in the UK.

A number of alterations during the 1980s set the scene for a new approach. First, the tradition of teaching hospitals being the only places which teach undergraduates came under pressure as increasing numbers of undergraduates required teaching. Many district general hospitals became involved in teaching. This also avoided the problems caused by shorter hospital stays and greater specialization, which made it difficult for students to see a broad cross-section of patients with common diseases.

It was also felt to be more important to concentrate on the process of carefully evaluating factual information, together with a range of intellectual and personal skills that would stand the test of time [401]. A number of medical schools had already considerably reduced the amount of basic science that students had to learn and this appeared to work well [402]. Students in some medical schools now spend a substantial part of their first years with general practitioners, occasionally visiting hospital when a patient they know is admitted.

The Newcastle experiment

This approach in Newcastle upon Tyne [403] has put greater emphasis on direct contact with patients. The behavioural sciences are used to guide students to understand the relationship between patients and the community in which they live. The teaching takes a life cycle approach which includes contributions from general practice, epidemiology and public health, child health, psychiatry, psychology and geriatrics. Each of these specialties is used to concentrate on a phase of the life cycle.

Students entering the medical school are divided into groups, each of which has a general practitioner tutor. The general practitioner recruits a number of families to the seminar group. At least one of the families will contain a woman due to have a baby within 3 months of the start of the project. Each family study is conducted by a pair of students, one man and one woman. The objectives of the project are for the students to observe and understand the background of the family they are working with, to understand the history of the pregnancy, labour and delivery, to observe the development of the newborn baby and the effect it has on the family and to understand the family's use of health and other services.

The students are also expected to observe and understand the family's interaction with society at large, in work, and in the community. Each pair of students reports back to their general practitioner tutor after the first few visits to their family and they have to write a full report on the project at the end of two terms, during which time they have kept in contact with the family. The family study project contributes 10% of the final mark in that year's examinations. At the end of the first term, halfway through their project, students are given advice by a specialist in population health (an epidemiologist) on how to describe the family in the setting of the wider population. They are expected to collect data from the family they are studying in order to look at a number of different facets, for instance, poverty and breast feeding or smoking and illness, and to combine these data with those discovered by the other students.

The intention of this part of their training is to examine the difference between medical facts taken from single patients and information derived from groups of people, on which diagnostic categories and treatment regimes are based. This part of the study also raises issues about the ethics and confidentiality of surveys and the opportunity is taken to discuss how such surveys can give biased results if some groups of people consistently refuse to take part and the problems that such data may create.

The data are used to help the students to put 'their own' family into the context of the population generally. The study findings are discussed in order to work out the best ways of providing medical care for different types of family and there is some discussion of how to use basic statistics.

The advantage of the family study is that it gives medical students, at an early stage, an introduction to communication skills and a concern about the lives and problems of the people that they are involved with. It also emphasizes home and background, allows students to see how epidemiological data can be used to put patients into context, and gives a broader view of how patients' problems fit into the community in which they live. This contrasts starkly with the traditional medical school where students still start their medical career with a systematic memorization of facts and develop considerable skill at dissecting, in minute detail, a corpse soaked in formalin.

Other schools give first year medical students experience of working in the community [404]. In this case, students work with people with chronic diseases. The general practitioners involved in the study were surprised to find that the students discovered a great deal of information about patients that was unknown to the general practitioners and considered by them to be of considerable use in the further treatment of their condition. It was therefore likely to improve the care that these patients received.

A review of 15 studies compared such innovative undergraduate teaching programmes with more traditional approaches. Schmidt, Dauphinee and Patel [405] found no difference in clinical competence, but a significantly larger proportion of graduates sought careers in primary health care and gave precedence to community based rather than hospital based care. It has been suggested that such relatively new approaches produce doctors with markedly better interpersonal skills, greater interests in continued learning and greater professional satisfaction in the work that they do [406, 407].

PROBLEMS OF THE APPROACH

The coordination of the whole programme is obviously much more difficult with students scattered throughout the community rather than kept together in one or a small number of central buildings. There is at present a huge shortage of teaching resources and skills in general practice. Much of what exists in hospital care may need to be transferred. It seems unlikely that this transfer of resources will be well received by the hospital based specialties, but this is likely to be mitigated by the increasing need for the consultants to work from community bases. The financial implications for university funding and the division of resources will have to be looked at in detail. Nevertheless, medical schools in a number of places have successfully made this change. As the dominance of the hospital reduces, such changes will be essential.

The first stage must be gradually to adapt the teaching curriculum towards integration of primary and secondary care together with epidemiology and possibly other support subjects, such as pharmacology and therapeutics. The actual teaching within these programmes will need to be considerably adapted but can be undertaken by the personnel already available for teaching. Central to the new approach will be the academic departments of general practice and epidemiology or public health. This will need to be gradually built up to the broader aims of, for example, the McMaster MD programme [408]. These objectives are:

- Knowledge: to acquire concepts and information to understand and manage health care problems.
- Skills:
  - Critical appraisal of clinical, investigational and published data.
  - Acquire, interpret, synthesize and record clinical information in managing the health problems of patients.
  - To identify areas of deficiency in own performance.
- Personal qualities: acquire authority to intervene in the lives of patients and acknowledge the obligation to act responsibly.

ADVANTAGES OF THE APPROACH

The McMaster programme has strengthened in two main areas since it began its teaching programme. There has been a development where public heath services attempted to bring together academic and service based public health. Another was the development of a centre dedicated to exploring ageing and health. This was aimed at bringing together the academic specialty of gerontology and service aspects, considering the special aspects of disease in old people.

Distance learning and team training

The developments I have been outlining will, apart from causing some difficulties with the traditional methods of teaching, also allow a number of opportunities for new ways of training. The change in emphasis from profession based approaches to problem orientated approaches (which is central to the way the McMaster programme works) means that much training can be given to mixed groups of professionals, instead of repeating the same facts to many different student groups.

Medical students, nurses, therapists and social workers will need to understand much more clearly than in the past the contribution that each should make. The simplest way of doing this is to amalgamate the common parts of their training. There is seen, at present, to be nothing extraordinary in training neurosurgeons and general practitioners together for the first 5 or 6 years. Many of the skills, knowledge and attitudes involved in the work of other professions is less remote from each other than the difference between those two medical professions.

Differences between the professions eroded

A number of groups, including the Welsh Health Planning Forum [409] and the Institute for Health Service Management [410], have suggested that the major divisions of medicine and surgery should give way to groups likely to be more relevant to the needs of the population when most patients are likely to need complex care crossing these barriers. In addition, it seems likely that purchasers will be keen to purchase care for a particular condition, which will include preventive and primary care elements, as well as curative and rehabilitation aspects, in order to specify more clearly the contracting process.

This fits in with the ideas contained in the strategic planning document *The Health of the Nation* [411] and the focus of the training suggested by the GMC. In future, there are likely to be more focused groups dealing with all aspects of a disease, such as cancer services discouraging smoking and offering surgery and palliative care services. Cardiovascular services will give dietary and exercise advice through to coronary artery surgery and exercise and psychological support as part of rehabilitation. Gastrointestinal services have been integrated for some time with combined medical and surgical units.

Such a change of emphasis will underline the great differences between the huge numbers of people requiring early preventive care or advice and the smaller number requiring inpatient care. The inpatient part will increasingly be seen as a small, if expensive, adjunct to the overall process of therapy for patients.

It is possible that the Royal Colleges, with their commitment to teaching medicine and surgery as different entities, may find it difficult to provide core courses for both in, for instance, cardiovascular medicine. They have shown a great ability to adapt in the past however, and such changes could be developed in quite a short time.

RETRAINING EXISTING STAFF

Retraining people already working in the health service is an excellent way to encourage change in the type of service that exists. Changes are no problem as long as one's position is safe. If this is not made clear they cause considerable anxiety among those involved. It is now generally realized that a flexible approach to training is essential for preparing for future changes. This has not been an obvious part of health service training in the past. Many professionals in the health service have been trained to follow rather rigid ways of doing tasks, despite the fact that patients very often vary greatly in their response to a set therapy.

The inability of hospitals to develop their own staff training was highlighted by a piece of research work by West and Anderson [412] who looked at new innovations in 24 major hospitals over a 6 month period. The data were checked by studying the minutes of all the senior management team meetings over that period, and where innovations had been set up they were checked in some detail.

Twelve senior managers and 16 occupational psychologists rated the innovations. They surveyed how great the consequences of the change would be, the extent to which that change was likely to alter the status quo, how new the change was, whether it was likely to be sidetracked into another path, the administrative efficiency needed to bring it about, patient care, and staff well-being. In the 24 hospitals, 184 innovations were introduced during the 6 month period, this ranged from 25 innovations in one hospital to three in another. The types of innovation were classified into four groups along two axes. The first axis had, at one end, an emphasis on flexibility versus control, the second related to internal versus external changes. Figure 11.4 shows the characteristics of the organizations which brought about innovations in each of the four categories.

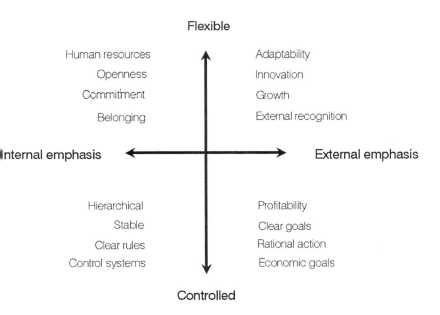

Figure 11.4 Characteristics of organizations that brought about innovations. (Reproduced with permission from [412].)

The most notable finding of this study was that the 'flexible, internally orientated' group was good at the development of training for its staff, but this group contained by far the smallest number of innovations, 12 in all. Half of the hospitals questioned did not have any innovations of this type, whereas only three hospitals failed to introduce innovations in the 'external orientation, control' group. This suggests that hospital managers, at present, are concerned with controlling the external and internal environment, not with developing their staff.

It also suggests that managers are keeping close control over the way that their people work and while aiming to care for their patients this care does not extend towards the staff working for the organization. It has often been suggested that caring organizations are likely to fail to care for those who work within them.

This is not to suggest that things are better in the community care parts of the health service. There has been no equivalent work done for community services. However, the organization of hospitals means that innovations for the development of the structures, hotel services, supplies and so on are likely to be given priority over the needs of staff. This appears to be less likely in the community where the structure of the service is not as rigid and where the needs of staff are more obvious.

There is also a long tradition about the way that hospitals work, with professional divisions and hierarchies. Interestingly this seems to stem from what, at first sight, seems to be the main strength that hospitals have – that staff of all professions and all grades are present in the building and, in theory at any rate, are accessible. It is possible that this grouping has led to some rigidity in the development of relationships between people and the development needs of the staff.

It is not usually difficult to instil new knowledge into staff who are about to undergo changes in their method of working, indeed much of the background knowledge that they already have may be relevant. New skills will be required in the move to community care including the ability to work in teams and to recognize what other people are capable of doing. In community work this may involve breaking down considerable prejudices. There are a number of professionals who have for many years had considerable suspicion and often antipathy towards one another.

General practitioners and social workers are good examples of this. The simplistic view is that general practitioners have a conservative, paternalistic approach to their profession and regard all social workers as having a Marxist tendency. This suspicion obviously has to be overcome at an early stage if the two groups are to work together successfully.

Team training

Most professions in the health service train separately from the others. The training of nurses, for instance, has been changing dramatically over the last 10 ears, yet few other professions are aware of these changes or of the new skills which nurses may have, especially in the areas of health promotion and interpersonal relationships. Working in teams means that a proportion of the skills possessed by one of the group needs to be shared with others; there needs to be intra-team training. If this is not the case then teams can become extremely cumbersome and the care they give very expensive. The good news is that this is reasonably easy to detect and the development of such teams is now reasonably well understood at a research level [413].

There are good opportunities for altering the methods of training that are being given at present. One reason for this is that government policy has required that more private and voluntary organizations have to be involved in the provision of services, particularly in the community. As a result, people with interesting and innovative ideas on the provision of services to patients are being brought into contact with health service and other professions.

GENERAL PUBLIC ATTITUDES

In the UK, there has been very little attempt nationally to explain the philosophy of moving mentally ill people into the community, despite the fact that such a move is likely to affect quite a large number of members of the public. The political approach, from both main political parties, has been that this is the right way to develop services and a vague feeling that it is believed to be better for patients. There is also a suggestion that developing community care is cheaper than using the existing services. As a result, Members of Parliament of both the main political parties seem to have strongly divergent views on the merits of the move to community care. It seems that the same individuals will at one time condemn the move as a means of cutting back services and at another promote such changes on civil rights and other grounds.

The policies have therefore been carried out so far with little informed public debate on the advantages to patients. The media appear to have left the public with a vague feeling that the whole process is a confidence trick on the part of the government to save money by releasing dangerous people into the community from locked wards. It may be British reticence, or ignorance, that makes health and other government ministers hold back from disclosing the philosophical basis for the change or even the suggestion that 'normalization', the central point of the underlying philosophy, has some virtue to it. There seems to be some embarrassment about taking an ethical stand on such issues. Perhaps this reflects a belief by successive governments that people will only act in their own best interests. There is, of course, always a downside to philosophy. A belief in normalization means that one also has to accept that in society mistakes will, on occasion, be made and mentally ill people will, albeit rarely, attack and harm members of the public or themselves. I believe that such issues need to be faced and discussed; but I do not need to be re-elected.

The Americans and Italians, both of whom put forward strong philosophical arguments for changes to community care for their mentally ill people, have developed a much more uniform structure for their care [414, 415]. Such an overview has meant, particularly in those two countries, a greater professional and lay interest and an interest in and awareness of the problems. This has not always been popular, but the debate has at least included a wider view than is presented, by the popular press in the UK, of 'mad' people on the rampage. The process of moving other services into the community is hardly discussed.

THE TOP OF THE HOUSE

The public in the UK, as in most democratic countries, do not have a great deal of direct power in shaping the details of policy on health or any other matters. Individuals feel they have little power to shape health policy by choosing a candidate at a general election. Individuals or a group of people are more likely to be able to alter the way that the local health authority provides its services. It may be thought of as the task of public health consultants to train the general public in how to have their voice best heard.

In the UK, the development of purchasing and providing in the NHS has been brought about at the same time as a change in the top management. The changes have not, in theory, been very dramatic, involving mainly a reduction in the numbers of people on the health boards and the addition of boards, complete with non-executive directors, to the trusts. It does bring up the topic of the best way to run large public organizations and how the public can, with assistance, have a voice in how the managers act.

It was made clear in Chapter 1 that the health service in the UK has never been run by elected representatives. Until the recent changes, ushered in by the NHS and Community Care Act 1990, the people who ran the health services locally were taken from three main areas: the local authorities; local eminent doctors or other professionals; and a mixture of the great and good, including prominent trade unionists. Often only the chief officer attended board meetings.

The problem was that the authority members would often represent a party or professional interest, rather than the interests of the health of the local patients or even the smooth running of the local services. The members sometimes appeared to be in a state of siege with their officers, with the latter attempting to hide the real consequences of actions inside complex technical language. Some members of authorities held pre-meetings, one of Labour the other of Conservative members to decide which way to vote.

Preventing the closure of hospitals which were no longer needed was often turned into a *cause célèbre* by one party or the other, in order to prove the inadequacies of the government of the day or of the party in the ascendant on the health authority. This has happened recently in my own area. A small health authority with a large number of members and few officers on its board has gone out of its way to destroy the general manager (until then an internationally renowned professor and leader in the field) at least partly to underline the short-comings of the national government.

This method of managing the health service has now mostly given way to a system of boards of directors, similar for both purchasers and providers. The boards are smaller with, usually, 10 members and a chairman. Five of the members are non-executive directors, chosen by the central government minister and five are executive directors – usually a chief executive, finance director, medical director, often a director of nursing and an administrative director, with a variety of titles. The non-executive directors are generally chosen for their business expertise. Some had previously been involved in the old health authorities. The theory was that the new authorities and trusts would be run much more along the lines of businesses, rather than as the traditional model of public service providers. The requirements of the internal market means that financial and managerial expertise, in particular, is especially prized. Most non-executive members of authorities and trusts therefore come from that type of background.

The emphasis on business expertise also means that a large number of the non-executives are directors of other companies and are therefore from a social stratum which is traditionally Conservative. This has led to accusations of bias from the Labour opposition and suggestions that they will bring their own people in once the government changes. It would be naive to suggest that the government was not aware of the advantages to it of using a group which was likely to be its supporters as non-executive members. There has always been a strong tendency for the government of the day to use its patronage to ensure its own supporters, rather than others, are put into positions of influence.

The health service trusts are, at present, at an early stage of their evolution, so it is not surprising that, at board level, there is a certain amount of euphoria. Apart from anything else many of the top trust appointments went to people who were in charge of hospitals or community units under the line management of the health authority general manager. The princes have become kings, without loss of blood, which is always greatly welcomed, by the princes at any rate. Nevertheless, there does seem to be a different ethos developing in the trusts.

The main positive difference seems to be that patients are seen as customers who can take their custom elsewhere and must therefore be reasonably satisfied with the care they get. It is true that patients have little direct control over the care they receive, but their general practitioners, especially those in fundholding practices, are thought to be more likely to take notice if a patient is given a bad time since the development of the internal market. In addition, trusts are aware of the move among health authorities to question their populations directly about the services they have used when deciding on two otherwise similar providers of services.

Services previously were provided by the officers of the authority who relied heavily on the view of the professionals working in the service, and worries about recent scandals to decide which areas of the service required more money.

This provided a somewhat paternalistic view of what patients needed and tended to be dominated by what was newly possible and in accord with the interests of powerful local hospital consultants, especially professors, and politicians.

There is still paternalism in the new system, just as there were some excellent attempts to avoid buying in new advances for their own sake in the old. However, there does seem to be some hope that the balance of advantage now lies with what works, in terms of making more people feel better, rather than what is scientifically interesting or the best way of keeping the vociferous quiet. The balance has swung a little towards trying to reduce the costs of a particular treatment or intervention or cutting out those which are not cost beneficial.

It will be necessary to train the public in these ideas, for the powers that shaped the old system (hospital consultants and politicians) are also expert at reaching and shaping public opinion. It is an urgent task for purchasers to point out the fallacies of this special pleading for pet schemes which cut across the strategic direction of the health authorities.

THE DEMYSTIFICATION OF HEALTH

The Alma Ata declaration [416] in 1978, reinforced the importance of primary health care as the basis for diagnosis and treatment in both developing and developed countries. Partly in response to that, and partly because of parallel pressures to those felt in developed countries, a number of developing countries have been concentrating their money on primary care services. This has often entailed transferring clinical activities from the wards, operating theatres and special units in hospital to local outpatient departments, day care units and home and community based services. This diversion of effort has also involved a strong health promotion aspect. Paine and Siem Tjam, in a book on the subject, make the central point: 'Such actions are beginning to break through the carapace of assured self containment with which many of the highly skilled, highly qualified professional staff of the hospital have too often surrounded themselves in the past' [1].

These ideas were not new in the 1970s. Paine and Siem Tjam describe a 'hospital without walls' programme set up 30 years before, despite considerable governmental and other opposition, in Costa Rica. The hospital still acts as a coordinating point for five health centres, five social security clinics and 46 health posts distributed throughout the area which it serves. It helps to develop health education and training for professionals in the community. A similar approach has been used in Nepal where a small district hospital is the central point for a large community organization. Health posts manned by paramedical staff serve the local population. The hospital resolutely refuses to develop tertiary or sub-specialty services, preferring to use its energy to develop the primary care facilities scattered around it.

Such approaches are not confined to developing countries. The North Central Bronx Hospital in New York, facing similar problems of large numbers of deprived people in the area, set up a Neighbourhood Family Care Centre in 1973 which attempted to treat families rather than disease. Specialist clinics in the hospital were phased out and replaced by five primary health care teams acting as independent units and responsible for all of the care for a particular group of families in the district. These teams included junior doctors, nurse practitioners, social workers, community nurses and family health technicians [417]. In another example, in Bihar, a particularly poor area of India, the only family hospital has 14 departments, one of which is run by a graduate of the College of Agriculture so that the health promotion message includes ways of improving agricultural efficiency.

It seems that in poor areas, where the pressure is great enough and where it is obvious that the main causes of ill health are social and therefore require social answers rather than bio-engineering answers, the hospital itself may be forced to break down in order to provide the social answers. There have been suggestions that the developed world could benefit from these ideas more generally, to help to meet increasing financial demands.

Halfdan Mahler, a previous Director General of the WHO, has suggested that medicine has progressively set up, whether consciously or unconsciously, a 'mystification of medical care' [418]. He mentions that, in order to maintain this mystification, the specialties continue to restrict the range of problems they consider themselves responsible for. He states that the gap between the maintenance of health care and medical care is becoming increasingly wide.

He also describes the restrictions set up on the information available about health care. Decisions that have been made by people in the health professions mean that the general population has become increasingly dependent on the holders of these mysteries. I have mentioned the medical mystification of most of our normal daily activities, which in the past were carried out for enjoyment: whether eating, sport or sex. Medicine has taken over the function religion had in the past as a regulator of these things and therefore a regulator of human life.

Mahler has suggested that people in public health medicine are the heirs of the great men of 19th century public health, like Chadwick, and should become social reformers like them. Their first job is to free the public from these mysteries by explaining them in detail. The second is to point out the extreme importance that other, more politically sensitive social conditions, such as housing, unemployment and poverty have on the health of groups and individuals within those groups. These are usually best summed up in terms of the wealth available to individuals.

Mahler describes the gross inequality in health expenditure in developing countries. In contrast to the past, most money is no longer spent on the wealthy but on an equally small proportion of the population which medical technology defines itself as being capable of dealing with. He mentions that this expenditure has never been proved to increase life expectancy or particularly improve the last few years of life. Despite this, most of the expenditure occurs during this period of existence for people in developed countries. There appears to be a trend towards defining the 'best' health care as that when everything known to medicine is applied to every individual by the highest trained medical scientist in the most specialized institution.

I have tried to point out in this book that there is now quite a strong counter-move. In the 20 years since Mahler wrote his article there has been some reaction against the mystification of health care, though not perhaps as much as he would have liked. Progress has been very slow.

Despite this, there has been some progress. Attempts been made to give people more knowledge of the origins of disease beyond simple ideas of germ theory and hygiene. Virtually everyone in developed countries knows that smoking is bad for health, but there is little idea of, for instance, the relative impact of cigarettes or the motor car on our health. In rare cases, the difficult decisions about what to do with scarce health money have been the subject of carefully organized public debate [419] but this is very rare and, as the people of Oregon discovered, expensive and fraught with political pitfalls.

There is some, though not at lot, of questioning of the place of the super-specialties in improving health. The effectiveness of cardiac transplantation, for instance, was questioned when many of the early patients died, but as more individuals survived the fuss subsided. There is little questioning about the central philosophy of developing such expensive treatments for such small numbers of people nor the right of the bio-engineering and medical professions to develop such approaches as long as they appear to work.

Once the system is mature and therefore capable of being tested against other approaches there is an argument that it is then established practice and cannot be changed. This circular argument has classically been exposed in the randomized controlled trials of coronary care units. The trials suggested that coronary care units did not work in terms of saving people from death. The cardiologists then cast around for other uses for them. They came up with the idea that coronary care units could reduce the amount of heart damage after a heart attack by giving drugs. This treatment can only, of course, be given in a coronary care unit.

Roberts [420], in 1952, suggested that no nation could afford to finance all the aspirations of its medical practitioners or satisfy the great expectations that these create in the minds of the people. He made the point that the increasing cost of ill health is due primarily and paradoxically to the advancement of medicine which is spurred on by the increasing speed of scientific discovery. If research wanted to achieve improvements in health on a global level it would stop being concerned with the investigation of the complex and subtle factors which underlie intractable diseases, such as multiple sclerosis, cancer of the breast and high blood pressure. These are insignificant problems in comparison with malnutrition and the persistence of infections and infestations. In Africa, Asia and Latin America half of all deaths occur in children under five [421].

THE PRESSURE FOR HOME CARE TO EXPAND

My thesis is that the move to community care is not something which has been planned, nor is it a 'movement' espoused by a minority of professionals or politicians for their own ends. It has professional advocates, working to their own agendas, certainly, and I am one of them. It still has a few, though less than there were, naive politicians who see it as a cheap option when they look at the enormous and increasing sums being spent on health care in hospitals. They cannot believe that there is not a cheaper way to do things. The costing of services for individuals, for instance, has shown, in my own district, that it costs £70 000 a year to keep some learning disabled individuals. It is hard to escape the thought that if we gave the person or their family half of that in cash they would surely be able to keep themselves at least as well as they are kept at present.

The move from hospitals to home based care follows a number of changes in society. Some of these are quite subtle and relate to suspicion of professional power bases, independence of and expectations of patients or customers, new possibilities for simpler treatments due to technological change, and the area of economics which is concerned with making any business or service flexible enough to meet new challenges. These pressures, I believe, are much more powerful than a lobbying group or a caucus with vested interests in the change.

Community care, at its most basic, is preferred over hospital care by the customers (the patients and their families) if all else is equal. However, there is not always a real choice if the disadvantages of the alternatives are overwhelming. For example, it is important that the difference between hospital and community care should be much more radical than simply trying get families to act as unpaid assistants in the care of their kin. The concept that a severely disabled person can be maintained at home with meals on wheels 5 days a week and a daily home help for 3 days is fatuous, but dies hard. The range and flexibility of the services and the specialist expertise they require is at an extremely early stage of development. A token stoma nurse or incontinence adviser will become involved in what will become serious issues in the next few years. Knowing the way the health professions have worked in the past, it will need specialist consultants, undergraduate training and a posse of postgraduate trainees to lift community services to anything like their real potential.

Power to patients

Treatment in the community is inherently based more on the patients' terms than on those of the doctors or nurses. We are the strangers in their home. This can, if we recognize it, allow a second facet to emerge: the ability of patients to help themselves much more than we allow them to at present. Options, such as retraining someone how to cook, rather than providing meals on wheels, training a young person to manage his or her own diabetes or epilepsy, is much easier in a home setting. Training relatives to help patients with their own physiotherapy after a stroke is a much more effective method of helping than giving them 20 minutes therapy once or twice a week in a crowded day hospital which looks like a third rate café on the Great North Road in the 1950s.

Simply treating someone at home may help, but it does not prevent professionals and carers from being patronizing, incoherent and uncommunicative. The changes needed to give good care outside hospital are as great as those changes which have been attempted for improving treatment and care inside hospital. The 'if you want me to use your surname you should be in BUPA' approach to service dies hard in the UK.

The future of general practitioner services

The structure of the health service in the UK is in a state of flux. It is unlikely that this will settle over the next 10 years or so. The fusion between health authorities and the family health services authorities, and the tendency for these to coalesce into larger groups, is accomplished in all but name. Purchasers for populations of somewhere near a million people will be in the odd position of having in them, but not quite integrated with them, most general practitioners, who are both purchasers and providers. General practitioner fundholding looks as if it will be extended, but it seems unlikely that all general practitioners will become fundholders over the next 10 years.

Special relationships between health authorities and non-fundholding general practitioners are likely to be set up so that general practitioners who are not fundholders can negotiate individually with health authority commissioners for a customized service for their patients. The future for consultants in public health medicine, the remaining doctors who are purchasers within the health authority, appears to lie with helping to draw together general practitioner requirements with the needs of the population. Their task will be to try to reconcile the two and then help to develop contracts with providers which contain the details of that compromise.

There is an increasing trend to identify subgroups of the population centred around groups of general practices and known in different places as localities, neighbourhoods or, in London, zones. These come in clusters of about 50 000 people. The aim is to identify groups which have special characteristics, for example, poverty, homelessness, high proportions of people belonging to ethnic minorities, or areas with a large numbers of elderly people. In this way it is hoped that commissioners can customize the service that they purchase to fit the needs of the local citizens. However, 50 000 people is too large a number to make much sense of this approach.

Such localities, in my experience, usually contain a broad cross-section of the different groups with special needs. My own view is that smaller groups, electoral wards for instance may have special needs requiring this special approach. Customizing services already happens at that sort of level, through the work of general practitioners. They are the most sensible grouping for specially customized services through the contracting process. It is likely that financial necessity and the integration of health authorities with the family health services authorities will result in a closer overview of the funds going to fundholding practices. It may be that general practice fundholding will become less popular as time goes on. Despite this, the general practice group is likely go from strength to strength as the basis for special contacts, whether or not fundholding is part of it.

A change of government could undermine the process of moving towards fundholding practices. The Labour party is, at present, committed to abolishing it. On the other hand, general practitioners will not easily give up the right to be able to specify the quality of the services they receive, or the specialists they wish to use, whether in hospital or in the community. The years of being 'second class citizens' and the possibility of, to some extent, reversing that process will be very dear to many of them. This may leave a future Labour government in a quandary, for they too are committed to the advancement of primary care. Whatever the future of fundholding, the relationship between general practitioners and specialists is likely to be considerably altered in future. General practitioners are aware that they have the power to enhance or diminish the influence of hospitals and the specialists within them.

There is a move, as mentioned in Chapter 6, for general practitioners to do some of their own needs assessment, to become their own epidemiologists. This process may develop but it seems unlikely that general practitioners will have time for purchasing, providing their own care, doing their own needs assessments, strategic planning and setting priorities. They are likely to leave the setting of priorities and decisions on which services are most effective to whatever remains of the commissioning authority, not least because it will be quite an unpopular task. Deciding that one service is a priority for new development will mean the withdrawal of finance from other services that appear not to come up to scratch – never a popular move.

The future relationship between the commissioning health authorities and the local authorities, especially social services, housing and education departments is not clear at present. In Wales, though not in England, local authorities are moving in the opposite direction from the commissioners of health services. The latter are developing into large commissioning agencies, whereas local authorities are grouping into small single tier units. These smaller groups contain about 1–2 000 000 people. These local authorities will contain the housing, education and social services, which will make the integration of those services easier. In a few areas, especially the borough of Hounslow in London, moves to integrate some or all of the health commissioning function with the local authority are being discussed. It remains to be seen if this will develop into a more widespread movement.

The future of trusts

Providers within the health services will all be trusts by 1996. In difficult areas this will be brought about by the takeover of the provider functions by the nearby trusts. The number of hospitals, the central theme of this book, is likely to continue to decrease, as will the number of purely hospital trusts. The move from hospital care, especially that in the London area responding to the Tomlinson report, will probably come about partially because of the necessity to avoid the overheads of a large number of buildings. This is now a big issue, for trusts are required to pay, in effect, a mortgage for the buildings they own. In the first instance, it seems unlikely that single specialty hospitals, particularly those providing geriatric and mental illness services, will survive the turn of the century. District general hospitals will follow within a further 10 years.

Some hospital trusts, in response to these pressures, will develop or combine with community units in their locality to provide their secondary services in concert with general practitioners or in small locality based modules. This has been well described in the recent report by the National Association of Health Authorities and Trusts [410] mentioned above. The report suggests that nine out of 10 surgical patients will be treated in day centres, developed in locally based units. Other more complex treatment will be gathered into regional centres. They suggest as few as 28 such centres in the whole of the UK, serving a population of about two million each. This would correspond roughly to the medical schools at present in the UK.

The central theme of the report is that care and treatment will be provided much closer to patients' homes than in the past. Primary and community services will take on the great bulk of the health services, and specialists will give their services in a wide variety of different settings. My own view is that 28 high tech centres may prove to be too many, especially if private companies develop diagnostic centres for pathology and imaging services. I would estimate about half of that number are necessary.

REGIONAL SUPER-SPECIALIST AND LOCAL UNITS

The present integration of family health services and district health authorities is likely to have an impact on general practitioners as providers. Those who are fundholding will be much more likely to purchase services from their own organization than from secondary care, and from secondary services in the community rather than from hospital based care. There are a large number of districts in the UK which are building small general practitioner inpatient units at present, known variously as community, neighbourhood or locality hospitals. It seems likely that these will take over many of the non-intensive care functions of district general hospitals, especially minimally invasive and day surgery and to provide a base for hospital at home services. In addition, many of the non-intensive casualty cases will be looked after in such areas, together with the moderately complex maternity cases.

Such places could provide the infrastructure for most home based rehabilitation services and all outpatient care. Good audiovisual and data links to the nearest super-specialist facility will be essential for the occasions when extra help is required or for unforeseen problems in patients who are too unstable to be transferred to the regional super-specialist unit. The highly specialized intensive and tertiary care is likely to be in small labour intensive units with very short lengths of stay.

PATHOLOGY AND OTHER SUPPORT SERVICES

It may well be that support services, such as pathology and imaging, will become specialist providers serving both the primary and secondary care market. They may on occasion be integrated with the specialist regional units, but equally may develop as separate organizations. Some of these services will become privatized. Other companies, based on the existing staff, may set up provider units giving a service to a very wide geographical area.

Improvements in the transport of data and automated testing systems will allow such units to be self contained. They are likely to be based in industrial sites rather than within a hospital complex, as access to goods will be more important than access to patients. They may produce specialist testing kits for the super-specialist centres and local units to perform emergency pathological work.

COMMUNITY TRUSTS

Community trusts will have particular problems with what is, for some of them, their central function, the community, child and adult district nursing services. They will have to be able to provide a service for general practitioners which is more cost effective than for them to employ their own nurses within the practice. There are several possible ways ahead for such trusts. The most satisfactory would be to expand into the provision of secondary services, using community based psychiatrists, geriatricians and paediatricians in the first instance. Later, other specialists, including day surgical units will join, and the development of hospital at home schemes will cover a high proportion of the acute general medical hospital work. They will also use these community based specialists to give direct advice to groups of general practitioners in their area in the prevention of disease and the development of shared care protocols. It is likely that nurse practitioners may find such work especially rewarding for they will be able to set up new services, rather than having to compete in the hospital based traditional service.

Other services community trusts develop may be subcontracted to hospital trusts, such as those which are particularly efficient at assisting with discharge from hospital. In this way the community trusts will enjoy the benefits of the popularity, with patients, of home based services, while not having to maintain hotel services.

FINANCES: ZERO BASED GROWTH

Over the next 5 years it seems unlikely that, in the UK at any rate, there will be any substantial growth in the amount spent on health care. It was mentioned in Chapter 3 that the UK spends relatively little on health care as a proportion of its gross domestic product, but it has been suggested that this is largely due to relatively low wages taken by the professionals, particularly nurses, compared with other countries.

Whatever the reason, due to its cost and in-built inflationary pressures, it may be that the present government and later ones will find it difficult to increase spending on health. There is a belief, though this is hard to prove, that the system of payment for health in the UK, coming directly from taxes, is a particularly efficient one. It seems unlikely that any government will be likely to go far in the direction of altering this over the next few years, if only because of the fear of increasing costs. There has already been grumbling about increased administration costs as a result of the division of the service into purchasers and providers. The increased number of managers will need to pay for themselves by greater efficiency. This has resulted in some government ministers restricting the further recruitment of managerial and administrative staff. This is always a popular political move and is not likely to be altered in the medium term.

CLOSING HOSPITALS

The closure of hospitals is always a difficult political pill to swallow. It appears that, at least in London, the reduction in the number of hospital sites is so entrenched in government planning that it is unlikely that all of the ancient and cherished institutions in the capital will survive the next 5 years. Having said this, I am aware that many carefully laid and apparently sensible plans have been completely overturned when they threatened the political stability of a particular minister or government.

I have a sneaking suspicion that the public, which individually has no great regard for going into hospital and does not, when the buildings exist as blots on the local landscape, seem particularly fond of them, changes its mind completely when there is a threat to the continuance of some of these ancient monuments. This is particularly extraordinary in the case of some hospitals which are in the memory of the people living near them and have formerly been known as places of horror – workhouses.

I strongly suspect that the sentiment for the retention of such places, despite all common sense, is often stirred up by the political opposition of whatever colour, which finds it a useful stick with which to beat the government. Many hospitals appear to be saved 'from certain closure' just before elections. Local professionals who have become used to working in the slum that the hospital has often developed into, fearing that their habits will be uncovered by closer scrutiny in future may also be in favour of such resistance.

It is one of the difficulties of developing and providing community based services that they are not, unlike the most innocuous Victorian workhouse, obvious to the naked eye. There is no large building for various members of the Royal family to open or to grace with their presence. There is no huge and inordinately expensive machinery for voluntary organizations to collect money for, there are no useful clusters of ill children for the local dignitaries to come and pat on the head at Christmas.

Hospitals have for many years represented symbolically the donation of health, by their masters, to a public which must learn to be grateful for it. Community based health services are much more easily made part of the population. They give the responsibility and to some extent the ability to achieve health, or to try to conquer disease, back to people themselves. This is not always welcome. When the result is that some odd looking people who have been locked up for 40 years or more because they were antisocial or abandoned or deaf are released onto the high street, there is even more outrage.

THE VOICE OF THE GENERAL PUBLIC

This raises a problem which has become very obvious since the recent changes in the UK health services: the problem of accountability and how it should be organized. Should the public, who pay for the service, have a say in what it provides or, more recently, what it should not provide? If it should have a say, how?

There are a number of approaches for letting the public have a say in the health service that they require, when the money is centrally financed either through direct taxation or through some kind of widespread insurance system. Aneurin Bevan in 1948 was resistant to allowing locally elected politicians to run the local health authorities. He was of the opinion that health services were too important to be subject to local party political squabbles and so set up a system in which the Secretary of State, the central government minister, decided who should run the health services.

As I have mentioned, until the recent changes (in 1991) these people tended to be chosen from the great and the good, locally. In other words, in the UK, there were quite a lot of local councillors of different political persuasions, often a number of highly placed doctors, and a number of trade unionists. I have a suspicion that Bevan had quite a strong regard for doctors and wanted them to have a considerable say in 'their' service.

I mentioned in Chapter 11 the sizable changes made in the management structure of authorities and trusts. The Secretary of State has chosen the chairmen and non-executive directors of trusts and health authority commissions from different backgrounds, compared with the previously existing boards.

Certainly the non-executive directors could not in most trusts or authorities pretend to represent a cross-section of the general public. There is no doubt that the political complexion of the non-executive directors tends to favour the right rather than the left wing of the political spectrum in the UK and this could not have been lost on the Secretary of State when the system was set up. Nevertheless, the ethos of paternalism does seem to have altered somewhat. Because of the competitive nature of the purchasing and providing system, particularly among providers, the deliberations seem to revolve around how best to provide an acceptable service to customers, that is the patients, within the money available.

I am concerned about the problem of the general public having a say in the way that health services develop. In the UK, at present, the most effective way is to depose the government of the day, and therefore the Secretary of State, in a general election. This is hardly a flexible way to bring about change. In the meantime it is to be hoped that the purchasers of health services will take seriously the need to be aware of what the general public wants and be able to modify their plans, to some extent, towards those desires.

The work must be much more positive than simply asking the local population what they want. The issues are often complex and technical and will need to be translated into understandable choices, without paternalism or propagandizing. This needs skill in communication and openness on the part of the commissioners, which has not been an obvious part of their make up in the past. Most commissions have attempted to get the views of the public or their patients about their plans in some way or other. But the central questions, about what values the local public hold, whether they prefer equity of access to high powered centralized facilities, whether some treatment services now should be disadvantaged for the development of preventive services in future, are not asked.

A simple and obvious example will give a flavour of the problems which the public should be involved in. Screening women for cervical cancer will save a few lives and give a very large number of women reassurance that they do not have the disease. Cervical cancer is rare and the screening money would be better spent, in terms of the number of lives saved, elsewhere. Do the public regard widespread reassurance as more important than saving a few extra lives? Health commissions will make these decisions, sometimes unknowingly, and make them without any recourse to the views of the population they are buying health services for. Indeed many health authority commissioners themselves have no stated set of values which would guide them into choosing one option or the other for cervical cancer. Most authorities try to get away with doing a bit of everything, while pretending to do everything to keep the public and their political masters quiet.

I have not mentioned the community health councils which, during this time, are supposed to have represented the general publics' view to the health authorities. They have not in my experience had any effect on policy or planning within the health service. They have been more successful at acting as advocates for individual patients who have fallen foul of the system.

BRINGING ABOUT THE CHANGES

Many of the changes described in this book have already happened or are well on the way to happening. Primary care is rapidly taking over most of the cure and care for children, leaving hospitals as supporters to the services provided. It seems likely that most community specialists in future will see their allegiance to a population group, whether it is called a locality or a neighbourhood, or the patients looked after within a group of general practices.

This process has been progressing for some years for learning disabled people. In fact the changes for this group are more radical because most of the routine care has moved out of health service hands to that of the social services. Health service people are still involved with clients with severe dependency or with people who are difficult to manage for other reasons. This involvement may be largely because of the higher staffing levels available and the expertise at dealing with disruptive people in health services units, rather than any intrinsic skill belonging to health.

The cure and care of mentally ill people is also well on the way to becoming a community based service, despite the difficulties. The main obstructions to progress appear to have been the estimated time scales suggested early on in the process. The development of acute intervention services based in the home have been consistently successful. It is likely to be only a matter of time before acute treatment in the home becomes the norm. Local, small and homely units can, and will, provide all long term care for mentally ill people.

Other services simply require the passage of time. Hospital at home schemes for elderly and terminal patients seem to be feasible and, triggered by the purchaser and provider split in the health service, seem to be developing in virtually every community based trust in the country. These are all eager to take on some of the lucrative inpatient therapy, presently the (expensive) mainstay of the hospital based trusts.

A new model

An important change has been an increase in public awareness of health services and of health in general. This partly arises from the alterations in the way that the health service is run and partly caused them. There has been a considerable spin off from the American health industry in that most of the issues, such as reducing dietary fat and running marathons, have been imported from the USA. Many of these have been health fads with little scientific evidence to back them up, but with enormous enthusiasm and a rapidly developed backing from industry, particularly selling those low fat spreads and sports goods.

This may seem a little cynical and it is certainly to be welcomed that people are taking the issue of health seriously instead of leaving it entirely to the professionals, as in the past. Much of the momentum to reverse the traditional awe in which professionals are held is maintained by the media in the UK which has realized that there is a great potential for scandal within health services and these scandals can sell newspapers or attract viewers. This contrasts with the USA where the financial advantages of doctors making mistakes was first realized many years ago by their lawyers.

It is essential that good straightforward non-propagandist information should be given to people to make sense of health issues. It is a failing of my own profession, public health medicine, that we have not taken on that task, despite being well placed to do so. It might be that in the next few years we may be forced to take up this important work by government policy. If we do not, other groups certainly will.

I have mentioned in the first five chapters of this book the pressures which have led us to the present time and the continuing pressures which will, I believe, continue to lead us towards a new shape for the health services. The interest of the public, the spotlight in which the health service is caught, may be the driving force for these pressures to keep their momentum. There is a public questioning of specialists which still swings between being obsequious and aggressive, but which is gathering momentum. There is a feeling that in Archie Cochrane's words [11], 'effective health care should be free for all', with emphasis on the word effective, and a more general understanding now among the public that much of medicine is inherited tradition rather than a carefully judged effective intervention.

Recent political changes have begun to increase the power of the general practitioners and raise expectations for the expansion of community services. A part of this, which I have not previously mentioned, is the rapid development of paramedically trained ambulance personnel. It can only be a matter of time before, using good communications and information technology, ambulance-men will be permitted to visit and leave at home patients who do not need admission to hospital.

Given further specific training it may be possible to ensure that patients who are unstable, for instance at home with a coronary or on the street after a vehicle accident, can be stabilized before being sent to hospital. All accident and emergency ambulances will carry paramedically trained crew members by 1995 which means that patients can be stabilized on the spot rather than having to go to a local emergency centre. This will allow a reduction in the numbers of hospitals taking emergency surgery in the future.

Deciding on the optimum use of staff

I have suggested that new financial and political pressures will push general practitioners to use different groups of staff as part of their primary care teams. This will increasingly involve working with, for example, social workers, specialist nurses, chiropodists, hearing technicians and voluntary organizations locally within their practice catchment areas, if not actually from the practice premises.

The community trusts will be under pressure from general practice in the field of the primary care services and this will result in an acceleration of the development of secondary care services, run by those trusts in the community. In particular they will, with social services, come to dominate long term care and rehabilitation care. They will, increasingly, be tempted to poach the traditional hospital based patients normally cared for in acute medical and geriatrics wards. The trusts will further develop hospital at home and small community based inpatient units.

Shared care

General practitioner purchasers will increasingly develop their own approach to chronically ill people based on a number of existing guidelines in the fields. People who require care with occasional back-up from secondary services, such as diabetic, epileptic and hypertensive patients, will fall into this category. It is increasingly likely that general practitioner fundholders will want to take on more of the work of caring for such people. They will develop joint agreements with hospitals or community based consultants and be guided by standard treatment protocols which take into account their own local requirements.

One of the difficulties that the health service has faced over the years has been a tradition of each profession keeping rigidly to its own area of knowledge and skill. As a result, junior members of staff are sometimes asked to undertake tasks which are better done by seniors and conversely very senior members of staff are involved in quite trivial tasks.

It should be said that this is a particular problem in the community where a large proportion of community nurses, because they are generally required to work on their own, are of a senior grade. The internal market will put pressure on providers to decide whether they can use fewer senior staff for doing specific tasks. In addition, there will be a careful examination of whether tasks undertaken in one place could be more cheaply undertaken in another. Tasks in the hospital may be better completed in general practice or in a patient's home. Much kidney dialysis is now being moved to home care. A proportion of minor surgery is increasingly done in general practitioners' surgeries. I have mentioned examples where ambulatory surgery has been done in general practitioner surgeries or small custom built units close to patients' homes.

In order to ensure that the right person is undertaking the right task a lot of work is being carried out to develop clinical protocols which give guidance as to where and who should be undertaking this work. A move towards community care will require a greater emphasis on disease prevention and health promotion. This will include the levels of self help and self care to be expected and will include details of the reasonable support which can be expected from family and other carers.

This in turn means that the emphasis needs to be changed from professionals doing things for patients to an approach where patients are helped and trained to help themselves. Another result of such work will be that consultants, while possibly having a small inpatient base, will be expected to move from place to place much more than in the past. There is a tradition that this is wasteful of a highly paid consultant's time, but it will be possible to complete some of the work using remote links by television or telephone.

Throughout this book it has been shown that the use of hospitals, as they are run at present, is extremely variable and generally inefficient. Far from being a high technology service, little of the care given us by the health service has a new technological aspect to it. There is an overemphasis on large complex pieces of machinery and large complex buildings, but these tend to be used poorly and for problems which are unlikely to be improved by their use. Over three-quarters of the costs of the health service go on staff rather than on technology. The most important reason for the development of community and primary care services as substitutes for hospital services is that, wherever this is practical and safe, patients prefer to be treated that way.

All of these changes are most likely to have an important and first impact on the district general hospitals throughout the country. It is likely, in the future, as now, that primary care teams will be the first point of access to patients who wish to receive help, whether health or social care. The teams are likely to include nurses, doctors (both general practitioners and some specialists), midwives, occupational therapists, social workers, chiropodists, counsellors and psychologists. It is likely that the local pharmacists will become involved. These teams could provide screening and assessment, where it has been shown to be effective, for those with both health and social difficulty. It is important that the teams should train together. This would be assisted by moving the primary focus for the undergraduate training of doctors, nurses and therapists in the first few years away from hospital into the community. Changes in the way that most professionals are being taught would fit in well with such a model. Most rehabilitation and long term care will be provided at that level.

Groups of primary care teams will probably have acute hospital at home services available to them and will be able to undertake much of the acute diagnostic and treatment work at present done by hospitals. A close relationship between the primary care team and the acute service provided by the hospital at home scheme would mean that, for instance, family members would receive social care and respite if that was needed when a person who was ill had become heavily dependent. The boundaries between the primary care teams and the specialists services will become increasingly blurred. The ability of these groups to work together will be assisted by clinical protocols.

Monitoring of the work done by the teams will increase in order to ensure that the strategic aims of the local health services are being taken into account. It may be that this will be part of the job of the consultants in public health medicine, working on behalf of the health authorities or even on behalf of the general practitioners. It is likely that some, at least, of this monitoring information will be published in increasing detail so that patients can choose between their primary care teams using relevant and well interpreted information. This, if it happens, will be the most important function of public health medicine.

The hospital services will concentrate initially on high technology treatment and trauma units covering quite large populations. The specialties within these units will be likely to cut across the traditional medical and surgical practice and will concentrate on combined medical and surgical treatment for such illnesses as cancer, heart disease or respiratory disease. It may be necessary to have some locally based inpatient beds near the primary care teams, in what may be described as neighbourhood or community or locality hospitals, but even these will, in time, be redundant.

It will gradually be realized that virtually all of the functions that even these small units have can be more cost effectively undertaken at home or in facilities akin to the UK nursing homes. The primary health care teams will of course require some kind of centre, if only to meet for coffee to enhance personal contacts between the teams. This centre may have a few beds in it for the cross-referral of patients and for training, but these will be very small in number and will accommodate patients only for very short periods.

WHO IS GOING TO DO IT?

Community health facilities in the UK centre around general practitioners. Generally, there is one general practitioner to every 1800 people in the population. The practices contain a number of practice nurses, managers and secretaries. A few practices have attached staff of one sort or another. The trusts with community responsibilities employ many district nurses, quite a few community psychiatric nurses, a few health visitors, and even fewer physiotherapists. Occupational therapists are also few in number and are divided into those who work for the health trusts and those who work for social services. There are some chiropodists, psychologists and speech therapists. There are a handful of community specialists: psychiatrists (often working both in the community and with their back-up inpatient beds), paediatricians and geriatricians. These all have relatively untrained ancillary staff to help them.

On the social services side there are social workers, home care assistants and their managers, who are relatively untrained and provide social support, increasingly more orientated to the disabled. There are people providing meals on wheels. A number of experimental ideas are being tried. Some voluntary groups provide a small number of services, especially for helping people after discharge from hospital and self help groups.

Some of these individuals are grouped together. Community mental health teams consist of nurses, social workers, psychiatrists and a scattering of other professionals with ancillary helpers. Their interrelationship with general practitioners and the rest of the general practice team varies from place to place. In some areas the community mental health team concentrates on secondary care, taking over outpatient, rehabilitation and rapid response acute care. In others they deal with the patients who general practitioners find difficult to manage. Most teams do a bit of both. A few groups have formed hospital at home schemes for the care of acutely ill people with specific diseases. Some have concentrated on the care of elderly people.

It is obvious that this scattered band of well meaning individuals, some of them organized, others not, will need to be considerably strengthened before they are capable of taking over the majority of routine health care. The problem, it seems to me, is that there has been little or no leadership in community care. One of two groups may lead the way in this.

The traditional approach is to employ specialist consultants in posts which are based in the community and allow them to develop teams around them with particular functions. The consultants, in other words, will take on this new task. The other possibility is that the new managers in the trusts, especially the community trusts, may take the lead in bringing together and training teams for specific purposes. Whichever it is, it is a most exciting task and is likely, in my view, to lead the way for the great majority of health services for the next generation.

References

1. Paine, L.H.W. and Siem Tjam, F. (1988) *Hospitals and the Health Care Revolution*, World Health Organization, Geneva.
2. Department of Health (1992) *Health and Personal Social Services Statistics for England*, HMSO, London.
3. Clay, R.M. (1909) *The Mediaeval Hospitals of England*, Methuen, London.
4. McKeown, T. (1976) *The Role of Medicine, Dream, Mirage or Nemesis*, Nuffield Provincial Hospitals Trust, London.
5. Abel-Smith, B. (1964) *The Hospitals, 1800–1948*, Heinemann, London.
6. Beveridge Report (1942) *Social Insurance and Allied Services*, Cmnd. 6404, HMSO, London.
7. BMA Advisory Panel (1967) *Health Service Financing*, British Medical Association, London.
7a. Ministry of Health (1968) *The Administrative Structure of Medical and Related Services in England and Wales*, HMSO, London.
7b. Department of Health and Social Security (1970) *The Future Structure of the National Health Service*, HMSO, London. In Wales there was a separate publication: Welsh Office (1970) *The Reorganization of the Health Service in Wales*, HMSO, Cardiff.
7c. Ministry of Health (1967) *First Report of the Joint Working Party on the Organization of Medical Work in Hospitals* (Chairman, Sir G. Godber), HMSO, London.
8. Bruggen, P. and Bourne, S. (1982) The distinction awards system in England and Wales 1980. *British Medical Journal*, **284**, 1577–80.
9. Advisory Committee on Distinction Awards (1993) Distinction awards, analysis by type of award, specialty and percentage distribution at 31 December 1992 – England and Wales. *Health Trends*, **25**, 80.
10. Ministry of Health (1962) *A hospital plan for England and Wales*, Cmnd. 1604, HMSO, London.
11. Cochrane, A.L. (1971) *Effectiveness and Efficiency. Random Reflections on the Health Service*, Nuffield Provincial Hospitals Trust, London.
12. Smith, R. (1994) Where is the wisdom...? The poverty of medical evidence. *British Medical Journal*, **303**, 798–9.
12a. Hasler, J. (1992) The primary health care team: history and contractural forces. *British Medical Journal*, **305**, 232–4.

13. Wolfensberger, W. (1972) *The Principle of Normalization in Human Services*, National Institute on Mental Retardation, Toronto.

14. Wing, J.K. (1982) Long term community care experience in a London borough. *Psychological Medicine Monograph Supplement*, No. 2.

15. Davies, B. and Challis, D. (1980) Experimenting with New Roles in Domiciliary Service, The Kent Community Care Project. *The Gerontologist*, **20**, 288–99.

16. Clarke, M., Clarke, S., Odell, A. and Jagger, C. (1984) The elderly at home, health and social status. *Health Trends*, **16**, 3–7.

17. Levin, E., Sinclair, I.A.C. and Gorbach, P. (1989) *Families, Services and Confusion in Old Age*, Gower, Aldershot.

18. Knapp, M. (1990) *Care in the Community. Lessons from a Demonstration Programme*, Personal Social Services Research Unit, Canterbury.

19. Boswell, D. (1988) *Care in the Community. A Comprehensive Local Mental Health Service in South Devon*, Open University Press, Milton Keynes.

20. Department of Health (1990) *Care in the Community, Making it Happen*, HMSO, London.

21. Raftery, J. (1992) Mental health services in transition, the United States and the United Kingdom. *British Journal of Psychiatry*, **161**, 589–93.

22. House of Commons (1990) *Public Expenditure on Health Matters*, Cmnd 484, HMSO, London.

23. Raftery, J. (1992) Mental health services in transition, the United States and the United Kingdom. *British Journal of Psychiatry*, **161**, 589–93.

24. Raftery, J. (1991) Social and community psychiatry in the UK, in *Community Psychiatry – the Principles* (eds D. Bennett and H.L. Freeman), Churchill Livingstone, London.

25. Doll, R. (1989) Demographic and epidemiologic trends today. *Arzneimittel Forschung*, **39**, 943–7.

26. Editorial (1990) Annual review. *The Economist*, December 1990.

27. Torrey, B.B., Kinsella, K. and Taeuber, C.M. (1987) An aging world. International Population Reports Series P-95, No. 78, US Department of Commerce, Bureau of the Census, Washington DC.

28. Benjamin, B. (1989) Demographic aspects of ageing. *Annals of Human Biology*, **16**, 185–235.

29. Morris, J.K., Cook, D.G. and Shaper, G. (1994) Loss of employment and mortality. *British Medical Journal*, **308**, 1135–9.

30. Gibbs, N.R. (1988) Grays on the go. *Time*, **131**, 66–75.

31. Callaghan, D. (1990) Must the old and the young compete for health care resources? *Neurosurgery*, **27**, 160–4.

32. Gavrilov, L.A. and Gavrilova, N.S. (1991) *The Biology of Life Span, a Quantitative Approach*, English edition, Harwood Academic Publishers, Switzerland.

33. Svanborg, A. The Götheborg longitudinal study. Ageing, living conditions and quality of life. Seminar. Norwegian Institute of Gerontology, pp. 56–63.

34. Feinleib, M., Kannal, W.B., Garrison, R.J. *et al.* (1975) The Framingham offspring study. Design and preliminary data. *Preventive Medicine*, **4**, 518–25.

35. Katz, S., Branch, L.G., Branson, M.H. *et al.* (1983) Active life expectancy. *New England Journal of Medicine*, **309**, 1218–23.

36. Manton, K.G. (1991) The dynamics of population aging, demography and policy analysis. *The Millbank Quarterly*, **69**, 309–39.

37. Bebbington, A.C. (1988) The Expectation of Life without Disability in England and Wales. *Social Science and Medicine*, **27**, 321–6.
38. Comfort, A. (1979) *The Biology of Senescence*, 3rd edn, Elsevier, London.
39. Davies, A.M. (19850 Epidemiology and the challenge of Ageing. *International Journal of Epidemiology*, **14**, 9–21.
40. Gumbel, E.J. (1958) *The Statistics of Extremes*, Columbia University Press, New York.
41. Hutchinson, G.E. (1978) *An Introduction to Population Ecology*, Yale University Press, New Haven.
42. Oliver, M.F. (1988) Reducing cholesterol does not reduce mortality. *Journal of the American College of Cardiologists*, **12**, 814–7.
43. Jennett, B. (1986) *High Technology Medicine, Benefits and Burdens*, Oxford University Press, London.
44. Rahmitoola, S.H., Grunkemeier, G.L. and Starr, A. (1986) Ten year survival after coronary artery bypass for angina in patients aged 65 years and older. *Circulation*, **74**, 509–17.
45. Campion, E.W., Mulley, A.G. and Goldstein, R.L. (1981) Medical intensive care for the elderly; study of current use, costs and outcomes. *Journal of the American Medical Association*, **246**, 2052–6.
46. Parno, J.R., Teres, D. and Lemeshow, S. (1984) Two year outcome of adult intensive care patients. *Medical Care*, **22**, 167–76.
47. Laslett, P. (1991) *A Fresh Map of Life. The Emergence of the Third Age*, Harvard University Press, Cambridge, Massachusetts.
48. Chow, R., Harrison, J.E. and Notarius, C. (1987) Effect of two randomised exercise programmes on bone mass of healthy postmenopausal women. *British Medical Journal*, **295**, 1441–4.
49. Wilkinson, R.G. (1994) Divided we fall. *British Medical Journal*, **308**, 1113–4.
50. Victor, C.R. and Vetter, N.J. (1986) A survey of elderly patients admitted to hospital for social reasons. *Archives of Gerontology and Geriatrics*, **5**, 33–9.
51. Ministry of Health Central Hospital Services Committee (1959) *The Welfare of Children in Hospital*, HMSO, London.
52. Committee on Child Health Services (1976) *Fit for the future*, HMSO, London.
53. Marks, L. (1991) *Home and Hospital Care: Redrawing the Boundaries*, King's Fund Institute, London.
54. Mair, A. (1972) *Medical Rehabilitation*, Scottish Home and Health Department, Edinburgh.
55. Tunbridge, R.E. (1972) *Medical Rehabilitation*, DHSS, HMSO, London.
56. Victor, C.R. and Vetter, N.J. (1988) Preparing the elderly for discharge from hospital, a neglected aspect of patient care? *Age and Ageing*, **17**, 155–63.
57. Townsend, P. (1979) *Poverty in the United Kingdom*, Penguin Books, London.
58. Ferguson, T. and McPhail, A.N. (1954) *Hospital and Community*, Nuffield Provincial Hospitals Trust, Oxford University Press, Oxford.
59. Garraway, H.M., Walton, M.S., Akhtar, A.J. and Prescott, R.J. (1981) The use of health and social services in the management of stroke in the community, results from a randomised trial. *Age and Ageing*, **10**, 95–104
60. Cay, E.L., Vetter, N.J., Philip, A.E. and Dugard, P. (1972) Psychological influences determining return to work after a coronary thrombosis. *Rehabilitation*, **81**, 27.
61. Lewin, B., Robertson, I.H., Irving, J.B. and Campbell, M. (1992) Effects of self

help post myocardial infarction rehabilitation on psychological adjustment and use of health services. *The Lancet*, **339**, 1036–40.

62. Preston, S.H. (1984) Children and the elderly, divergent paths for America's dependents. *Demography*, **21**, 436–57.
63. Estes, C.L. and Swan, J.H. (eds) (1993) *The Long Term Care Crisis*, Sage Publications, London.
64. Jamieson, A. (ed.) (1991) Home care provision and allocation, in *Home Care for Older People in Europe: Policies and Practices*, Oxford University Press, Oxford.
65. Jamieson, A. (1993) Home care in old age, a lost cause? *Journal of Health Politics, Policy and Law*, **17**, 879–98.
66. Bennett, C.L. (1993) Health care in Austria. *Journal of the American Medical Association*, **269**, 2789–94.
67. Malcolm, L. (1990) Service management, New Zealand's solution to the problems of quality assurance and financial control. *Cahiers de Sociologie et de Démographie Médicin*, **30**, 363–79.
68. Ogbu, O. and Gallagher, M. (1992) Public expenditures and health care in Africa. *Social Science and Medicine*, **34**, 615–24.
69. Binstock, R.H. and Post, S.G. (eds) (1991) *Too Old for Health care. Controversies in Medicine, Law, Economics and Ethics*, Johns Hopkins University Press, Baltimore, Maryland.
70. Charny, M.C., Lewis, P.A. and Farrow, S.C. (1989) Choosing who shall not be treated in the NHS. *Social Science and Medicine*, **28**, 1331–8.
71. World Bank (1993) *World Development Report 1993*, Oxford University Press, Oxford.
72. Illich, I. (1977) *Limits to Medicine*, Penguin Books, London.
73. World Health Organization (1978) *Primary Health Care*, Alma Ata. Health for All Series No 1. WHO, Geneva.
74. World Bank (1993) *World Development Report 1993. Investing in Health*, Oxford University Press, Oxford.
75. Office of Health Economics (1989) *Compendium of Health Statistics*, 7th edn, Office of Health Economics, London.
76. Blank, R.H. (1991) Rationing medicine, hard choices in the 1990s. *The American Journal of Gastroenterology*, **87**, 1076–84.
77. Charny, M.C., Lewis, P.A. and Farrow, S.C. (1989) Choosing who shall not be treated in the NHS. *Social Science and Medicine*, **28**, 1331–8.
78. Welsh Health Planning Forum (1989) *Local Strategies for Health: a New Approach to Strategic Planning*, Welsh Office, NHS Directorate, Cardiff.
79. Welsh Health Planning Forum (1992) *Health and Social Care 2010*, Welsh Office, Cardiff.
80. Fertig, A., Roland, M., King, H. and Moore, T. (1993) Understanding variation in rates of referral among general practitioners, are inappropriate referrals important and would guidelines help to reduce rates? *British Medical Journal*, **307**, 1467–70.
81. Culyer, A. and Brazier, J. (1988) *Alternatives for Organising the Provision of Health Services in the UK*, IHSM, London.
82. Department of Health (1989) *Working Paper No 1. Self Governing Hospitals*, HMSO, London.
83. Harrison, S., Hunter, D. and Pollitt, C. (1990) *The Dynamics of British Health Policy*, Unwin Hyam, London.
84. Ovretveit, J. (1993) Purchasing for health gain. The problems and prospects for

purchasing for health gain in the 'managed markets' of the NHS and other European health systems. *European Journal of Public Health*, **3**, 77–84.

85. Townsend, P. and Davidson, N. (eds) (1992) *Inequalities in Health*, Penguin, London.

86. Gupta, S. (1991) *The Mental Health Problems of Migrants: Report from Six European Countries*, WHO Regional Office for Europe, Copenhagen.

87. Robinson, R. and Le Grand, J. (eds) (1994) *Evaluating the NHS Reforms*, King's Fund Institute, London, pp. 24–53.

88. Glennerster, H., Matsaganis, M. and Owens, P. (1992) *A Foothold for Fundholding*, King's Fund Institute, London.

89. Harrison, S. (1991) Working the markets, purchaser/provider separation in English health care. *International Journal of Health Services*, **21**, 625–35.

90. Balinsky, W. and Starkman, J. (1987) The impact of diagnostic related groups on the health care industry. *Health Care Management Review*, **12**, 61–74.

91. Wilkinson, R.G. (1994) Divided we fall. *British Medical Journal*, **308**, 1113–4.

92. Vetter, N.J., Cay, E.L., Philip, A.E. and Strange, R.C. (1977) Anxiety on admission to a coronary care unit. *Journal of Psychosomatic Research*, **21**, 73–8.

93. Vetter, N.J. and Julian, D.G. (1975) Comparison of an arrhythmia computer and conventional monitoring in a coronary care unit. *The Lancet*, **1**, 1151–4.

94. McGinnis, J.M. (1989) National priorities in disease prevention. *Issues in Science and Technology*, **5**, 46–52.

95. Schramm, C.J. (1984) Can we solve the hospital cost problem in our democracy? *New England Journal of Medicine*, **311**, 729–32.

96. Herdman, R.C., Wagner, J.L., Wolfe, L. *et al.* (1993) Health technology and health reform. *Cancer Investigation*, **11**, 337–44.

97. Noz, M.E., Erdman, W.A. and Maguire, G.Q. (1986) Local area networks in an imaging environment. *Critical Reviews in Medical Information*, **1**, 81–133.

98. Hutton, J. and Williams, A.H. (1988) Cost effectiveness analysis of diagnostic technology, in *Health Care Systems and Factors. Fourth International Society for System Science in Health Care* (eds G. Durn, R. Engelbrecht, C.D. Flagle and W. Van Eimeren), Masson, Paris, pp. 493–6.

99. Shuman, W.P. (1988) The poor quality of early evaluations of MR imaging, a reply. *American Journal of Radiology*, **151**, 857–8.

100. Kent, D.L. and Larson, E.B. (1988) Magnetic resonance imaging of the brain and spine – is clinical efficiency established after the first decade? *Annals of Internal Medicine*, **108**, 402–24.

101. Cooper, L.S., Chalmers, T.C., McCally, M. *et al.* (1988) The poor quality of early evaluations of magnetic resonance imaging. *Journal of the American Medical Association*, **259**, 3277–80.

102. Friedman, P.J. (1988) The early evaluations of MR imaging. *American Journal of Radiology*, **15**, 860–1.

103. Teasdale, G.M., Hadley, D.M. and Lawrence, A. (1989) Comparison of magnetic resonance imaging and computed tomography in suspected lesions in the posterior cranial fossa. *British Medical Journal*, **299**, 349–55.

104. Dixon, A.K., Southern, J.P., Teale, A. *et al.* (1991) Magnetic resonance imaging of the head and spine; effective for the clinician or the patient? *British Medical Journal*, **302**, 78–82.

105. Centre for Health Economics (1990) *Economic Evaluation of the Clinical*

Application of MR Imaging. Final Report, MRC Special Project Grant, MRC, London.

106. Warner, M.M., Pugh, S., Riley, C. and Rhodes, J. (1993) *Blurring the Boundaries. The Future of Hospital and Primary Care*, Welsh Health Planning Forum, Cardiff.
107. Amara, R. (1988) *Looking Ahead at American Healthcare*, Healthcare Information Center, McGraw-Hill, Washington DC.
108. Office of Technology Assessment (1984) *Commercial Biotechnology: an International Analysis*, US Government Printing Office, Washington DC.
109. Holtzman, N.A. (1989) *Proceed with Caution. Predicted Genetic Risks in the Recombinant DNA Era*, Johns Hopkins University Press, Baltimore.
110. Banta, H.D. (1990) Future health care technology and the hospital. *Health Policy*, **14**, 61–73.
111. Editorial (1990) Biotechnology and the drug industry. *British Medical Journal*, **300**, 146–7.
112. Office of Technology Assessment (1983) *Assistive Devices for Severe Speech Impairments. Health Technology Case Study 26*, US government Printing Office, Washington DC.
113. Office of Technology Assessment (1982) *Technology and Handicapped People*, US Government Printing Office, Washington DC.
114. Blackshear, P.J. (1985) Implantable infusion pumps, clinical applications. *Methods in Enzymology*, **112**, 520–30.
115. Editorial (1988) Twenty five years of coronary care. *The Lancet*, **2**, 830–1.
116. Keighley, M.R.B. and Williams, N.S. (1993) *Surgery of the Anus, Rectum and Colon*, WB Saunders, London.
117. Javitt, J.C., Canner, M.K. and Sommer, A. (1989) Cost effectiveness of current approaches to the control of retinopathy in Type I diabetics. *Ophthalmology*, **96**, 255–64.
118. Forrester, J.S., Eigler, N. and Litvak, F. (1991) Interventional cardiology. The decade ahead. *Circulation*, **84**, 942–4.
119. Brooks, L. and Black, M. (1994) Local delivery. *Health Service Journal*, **104**, 33–5.
120. Madhok, R., Bhopal, R.S. and Ramaiah, R.S. (1992) Quality of hospital service, a study comparing Asian and non Asian patients in Middlesbrough. *Journal of Public Health Medicine*, **14**, 271–9.
121. Smith, C. (1992) Validation of a patient satisfaction system in the United Kingdom. *Quality Assurance in Health Care*, **4**, 171–7.
122. Donabedian, A. (1980) *The Definition of Quality and Approaches to its Assessment. Explorations in Quality Assessment and Monitoring. Vol. 1*, Health Administration Press, Ann Arbor, MI.
123. Vuori, H. (1987) Patient satisfaction – an attribute or indicator of the quality of care? *Quality Review Bulletin*, **13**, 106–9.
124. Salvage, A.V. (1986) *Attitudes of the Over 75s to Health and Social Services*, Research Team for the Care of the Elderly, Cardiff.
125. Borough of Haringey (1985) A study of the awareness of Haringey residents of the social services department and general attitudes towards social services. London Borough of Haringey, Social Services Department, London.
126. Snider, E.L. (1980) Awareness and Use of Health Services by the Elderly: A Canadian Study. *Medical Care*, **18**, 1177.
127. Connelly, N. and Goldberg, T. (1979) Looking at meals on wheels. *Community Care*, **26**, 20–3.

128. Airey, C. and Jowell, R. (1984) *British Social Attitudes: the 1984 Survey*, Gower, London.
129. Bowling, A. and Salvage, A.V. (1984) *Prevention of Institutional Admission in City and Hackney*, Centre for the Study of Primary Care, London.
130. Thompson, C. and West, P. (1984) The public appeal of sheltered housing. *Ageing and Society*, **4**, 305–26.
131. Salvage, A.V., Vetter, N.J. and Jones, D.A. (1988) Attitudes to hospital care among a community sample of people aged 75 and older. *Age and Ageing*, **17**, 270–4.
132. Kennedy, R.D. and Acland, S.M.S. (1976) Attitudes of the elderly and their relatives to geriatric admission. *Health Bulletin*, **34**, 320–4
133. McAlpine, C.J. and Wight, Z.J. (1982) Attitudes and anxieties of elderly patients on admission to a geriatric assessment unit. *Age and Ageing*, **11**, 35–41.
134. Pica-Furey, W. (1993) Ambulatory surgery – hospital based vs freestanding. *AORN Journal*, **57**, 1119–27.
135. Brown, P. (1985) *The Transfer of Care*, Routledge, London.
136. Knapp, M. (1990) *Care in the Community. Lessons from a Demonstration Programme*, Personal Social Services Research Unit, Canterbury.
137. Corrigan, P.W. (1990) Consumer satisfaction with institutional and community care. *Community Mental Health Journal*, **26**, 151–65.
138. Gillig, P., Grubb, P., Kruger, P. *et al.* (1990) What do psychiatric emergency patients really want and how do they feel about what they get? *Psychiatric Quarterly*, **61**, 189–96.
139. Tybjerg, J., Boller, S., Valbak, K. and Lindhardt, A. (1990) Psychiatric hospitalizations evaluated by patients. *The International Journal of Social Psychiatry*, **36**, 163–71.
140. Eichorn, S. (1985) A hospital humanises patient care. *Hospital Forum*, **28**, 55–7.
141. Piersma, H. (1983) Program evaluation using a public opinion survey, one hospital's experience. *The Psychiatric Hospital*, **14**, 171–6.
142. Sullivan, C.W. and Yudelowitz, I.S. (1991) Staff and patients, divergent views of treatment. *Perspectives in Psychiatric Care*, **27**, 26–30.
143. Corrigan, P.W. (1990) Consumer satisfaction with institutional and community care. *Community Mental Health Journal*, **26**, 151–65.
144. McEvoy, J., Aond, J., Wilson, W. *et al.* (1981) Measuring chronic schizophrenic patients' attitudes towards their illness and treatment. *Hospital and Community Psychiatry*, **32**, 856–7.
145. Goldstein, R.H., Racy, J., Dressler, D.M. *et al.* (1972) What benefits patients? *Psychiatric Quarterly*, **46**, 49–80.
146. Distephano, M., Pryer, M. and Garrison, J. (1980) Attitudinal, demographic and outcome correlates of clients' satisfaction. *Psychological Reports*, **45**, 287–90.
147. Perring, C. (1992) The experience and perspectives of patients and care staff of the transition from hospital to community-based care, in *Psychiatric Hospital Closure. Myths and Realities* (ed. S. Ramon), Chapman & Hall, London, pp. 122–68.
148. Robertson, J. (1958) *Young Children in Hospital*, Tavistock, London.
149. Rutter, M. (1972) *Maternal Deprivation Reassessed*, Penguin, London.
150. Quinton, D. and Rutter, M. (1976) Early hospital admission and later disturbances of behaviour. *Developmental Medicine and Child Neurology*, **18**, 447–59.
151. Cleary, J., Gray, O.P., Hall, D.J. *et al.* (1986) Parental involvement in the lives of children in hospital. *Archives of Disease in Childhood*, **61**, 779–87.

152. Andrews, M.M. and Nielson, D.W. (1988) Technology dependent children in the home. *Pediatric Nursing*, **14**, 111–4.
153. Department of Health (1989) *Working for Patients*, Cmnd 555, HMSO, London.
154. While, A.E. (1992) Consumer views of health care, a comparison of hospital and home care. *Child, Health, Care and Development*, **18**, 117–28.
155. Attwell, J.D. and Gow, M.A. (1985) Paediatric trained district nurse in the community, expensive luxury or economic necessity? *British Medical Journal*, **231**, 227–9.
156. Jackson, R.H. (1978) Home care for children. *Journal of Maternal and Child Health*, **3**, 96–100.
157. Couriel, J.M. and Davies, D. (1988) Costs and benefits of a community special care baby service. *British Medical Journal*, **296**, 1043–6.
158. Connell, F.A., Day, R.W. and LoGerfo, J.P. (1981) Hospitalization of Medicaid children, analysis of small area variations in admission rates. *American Journal of Public Health*, **71**, 606–13.
159. Wennberg, J. and Kim, S.Y.S. (1977) Common uses of hospitals. A look at Vermont, in *Harvard Child Health Project. Vol. 2*, Ballinger, Cambridge, MA, pp. 353–82.
160. Kemper, K.J. (1988) Medically inappropriate hospital use in a pediatric population. *New England Journal of Medicine*, **318**, 1033–7.
161. Perrin, J.M., Homer, C.J., Donald, M.P.H. *et al.* (1989) Variations in rates of hospitalization of children in three urban communities. *New England Journal of Medicine*, **320**, 1183–7.
162. Wright, K.G., Cairns, J.A. and Snell, M.C. (1981) *Costing care*, Social Services Monographs, Research in Practice, Community Care, Sheffield.
163. Counsel and Care (1992) *From Home to a Home*, Counsel and Care, London.
164. Warren, M.W. (1946) Care of the chronic aged sick. *The Lancet*, **1**, 841–3.
165. Mather, H.G., Morgan, D.C., Pearson, N.G. *et al.* (1976) Myocardial infarction, a comparison between home and hospital care for patients. *British Medical Journal*, **1**, 925–9.
166. Langhorne, P., Williams, B.O., Gilchrist, W. and Howie, K. (1993) Do stroke units save lives? *The Lancet*, **342**, 395–8.
167. Wade, D.T., Langton-Hewer, R., Skilbeck, C.E. *et al.* (1985) Controlled trial of a home care service for acute stroke patients. *The Lancet*, **1**, 323–6.
168. Adler, M.W., Waller, J.J., Creese, A. and Thorne, S.C. (1978) Randomised controlled trial of early discharge for inguinal hernia and varicose veins. *Journal of Epidemiology and Community Health*, **32**, 136–42.
169. Gerson, L.W. and Collins, J.F. (1976) A randomized controlled trial of home care, clinical outcome for five surgical procedures. *The Canadian Journal of Surgery*, **19**, 519–23.
170. Torres, A. and Reich, M.R. (1989) The shift from home to institutional childbirth: a comparative study of the United Kingdom and The Netherlands. *International Journal of Health Services*, **19**, 405–14.
171. Maternity Services Advisory Committee (1984) *Maternity Care in Action. A Guide to Practice and a Plan for Action*, HMSO, London.
172. Tew, M. (1979) The safest place of birth, further evidence. *The Lancet*, **1**, 1388–90.
173. MacVicar, J., Dobbie, G., Owen-Johnstone, L. *et al.* (1993) Simulated home delivery in hospital, a randomised controlled trial. *British Journal of Obstetrics and Gynaecology*, **100**, 316–23.

174. Thorogood, M., Mann, J., Appleby, P. and McPherson, K. (1994) Risk of death from cancer and ischaemic heart disease in meat and non-meat eaters. *British Medical Journal*, **308**, 1667–71.

175. Larson, R. (1979) Thirty years of research on the subjective well-being of older Americans. *Journal of Gerontology*, **33.1**, 109–25.

176. Hofstetter, C.R., Sallis, J.F. and Hovell, M.F. (1990) Some dimensions of self-efficacy, analysis of theoretic specificity. *Social Science and Medicine*, **31**, 1051–6.

177. Bandura, A. (1977) Self efficacy, towards a unifying theory of behaviour change. *Psychological Review*, **84**, 191–215.

177a. Vetter, N.J., Charny, M., Lewis, P.A. *et al.* (1991) Health, fatalism and age in relation to lifestyle. *Health Visitor*, **64**, 191–4.

178. Lewis, P.A. and Charny, M. (1987) The Cardiff Health Survey: teaching survey methodology by participation. *Statistics in Medicine*, **6**, 869–74.

179. Charny, M. and Lewis, P.A. (1987) Does health knowledge affect eating habits? *Health Education Journal*, **46**, 172–6.

180. Anon (1988) *Promoting Health Among Elderly People*, King Edward's Hospital Fund for London, London.

181. United States Department of Health and Human Services, Public Health Services (1980) *Promoting Health: Preventing Disease*, Government Printing Office, Washington DC.

182. Kennedy, R.D. and Acland, S.M.S. (1976) Attitudes of the elderly and their relatives to geriatric admission. *Health Bulletin*, **34**, 320–4.

183. Harris, L. (1975) *The Myth and Reality of Aging in America*, National Council on the Aging, Washington DC.

184. Goldmann, R. and Goldmann, J. (1982) *Children's Sexual Thinking*, Routledge and Kegan Paul, London.

185. Rabbitt, P. (1981) Talking to the old. *New Society*, 22 Jan, 140–1.

186. Editorial (1975) Smoking in The Elderly, *British Medical Journal*, **2**, 607–8.

187. Gray, M. (ed.) (1985) *Prevention of Disease in the Elderly*, Churchill Livingstone, London.

188. WHO Advisory Group (1986) *The Effectiveness of Health Promotion for the Elderly*, WHO, Hamilton, Canada.

189. Kane, R.L. (1988) Empiric approaches to prevention in the elderly: are we promoting too much?, in *Health Promotion and Disease Prevention in the Elderly* (eds R. Chernoff and D.A. Lipschitz), Raven Press, New York, p. 164.

190. Vetter, N.J. and Ford, D. (1990) Smoking Prevention Among People Aged 60 and Over: A Randomised Controlled Trial. *Age and Ageing*, **19**, 164–8.

191. Audit Commission (1992) *Lying in Wait: the Use of Medical Beds in Acute Hospitals*, HMSO, London.

192. Rabins, P.V., Mace, N.L. and Lucas, M.J. (1982) The impact of dementia on the family. *Journal of the American Medical Association*, **248**, 333–5.

193. Seltzer, M.M., Litchfield, L.C., Kapust, L.R. and Mayer, J.B. (1992) Professional and family collaboration in case management, a hospital based replication of a community based study. *Social Work in Health Care*, **17**, 1–22.

194. Seltzer, M.M., Ivry, J. and Litchfield, L.C. (1987) Family members as case managers, partnership between the formal and the informal support networks. *The Gerontologist*, **27**, 722–8.

195. Anderson, P., Meara, J., Brodhurst, S. *et al.* (1988) Use of hospital beds, a cohort study of admissions to a provincial teaching hospital. *British Medical Journal*, **297**, 910–2.

196. Restuccia, J.D., Gertman, P.M., Dayno, S.J. *et al.* (1984) A comparative analysis of appropriateness of hospital use. *Health Affairs*, **3**, 130–8.

197. Torrance, N., Lawson, J.A.R., Hogg, B. and Knox, J.D.G. (1972) Acute admissions to medical beds. *Journal of the Royal College of General Practitioners*, **22**, 211–9.

198. Lagoe, R.J. (1986) Differences in hospital discharge rates. A community based analysis. *Medical Care*, **24**, 868–72.

199. Gertman, P.M. and Restuccia, J.D. (1981) The appropriateness evaluation protocol, a technique for assessing unnecessary days of hospital care. *Medical Care*, **19**, 855–71.

200. Rosser, R.M. (1976) Reliability and application of clinical judgment in evaluating the use of hospital beds. *Medical Care*, **14**, 39–47.

201. Restuccia, J.D. (1982) The effect of concurrent feedback in reducing inappropriate hospital utilization. *Medical Care*, **20**, 46–62.

201a. Vetter, N.J., Jones, D.A. and Victor, C.R. (1986) A health visitor affects the problems others do not reach. *The Lancet*, **2**, 30–2.

202. Davies, B. and Challis, D. (1980) Experimenting with new roles in domiciliary service: the Kent Community Care Project. *The Gerontologist*, **20**, 288–99.

203. Kane, R.A. (1990) Case management and assessment of the elderly, in *Improving the Health of Older People* (eds R.L. Kane, J. Grimley Evans and D. Macfadyen), Oxford University Press, Oxford, pp. 398–416.

204. Frankfather, D.L., Smith, M.J. and Caro, F.G. (1981) *Family Care of the Elderly: Public Initiatives and Private Obligations*, Heath, Lexington, MA.

205. Seltzer, M.M., Simmons, K., Ivry, J. and Litchfield, L. (1984) Family agency partnerships, case management of services for the elderly. *Journal of Gerontological Social Work*, **7**, 57–71.

206. Hicks, B., Raisz, H., Segal, J. and Doherty, N. (1981) The triage experiment in coordinated care for the elderly. *American Journal of Public Health*, **71**, 991–1003.

207. Yordi, C.L. and Waldeman, J. (1985) A consolidated model of long term care, service utilisation and cost impacts. *The Gerontologist*, **25**, 389–97.

208. Bird, K.T. (1972) Cardiopulmonary frontiers, quality healthcare via interactive television. *Chest*, **61**, 204–5.

209. Watson, D.S. (1989) Telemedicine. *The Medical Journal of Australia*, **151**, 62–71.

210. Horowitz, L.N. (1989) Ventricular arrhythmias, control of therapy by Holter monitoring. *European Heart Journal*, **10**, Suppl E, 53–60.

211. Tomlinson, B. (1992) *Report of the Inquiry into London's Health Service, Medical Education and Research*, HMSO, London (The Tomlinson Report).

212. Department of Health (1993) *Making London Better*, Department of Health, London.

213. Anderson, H.J. (1986) High technology services help cut lengths of stay, save money. *Modern Healthcare*, **16**, 90–2.

214. Marks, L. (1991) *Home and Hospital Care: Redrawing the Boundaries*, King's Fund Institute, London.

215. Frasca, C. and Christy, M.W. (1986) Assuring continuity of care through a hospital based home health agency. *Quality Review Bulletin*, **12**, 167–71.

216. Wynn, L., Dingle, J., Hogan, D. *et al.* (1989) *Before and After the New Brunswick Extra Mural Hospital, an Analysis of Traditional Hospital Utilization*, Dalhousie University Medical School, Halifax, Nova Scotia.

217. Anand, J.K. and Pryor, G.A. (1989) Hospital at home. *Health Trends*, **21**, 46–8.

218. Ferguson, G. (1987) The New Brunswick extra mural hospital, a Canadian hospital at home. *Journal of Public Health Policy*, **8**, 561–70.

219. King Edward's Hospital Fund for London (1973) *Accounting for Health. Report of a Working Party on the Application of Economic Principles to Health Service Management*, King's Fund, London.

220. Hedrick, S.C. and Inui, T.S. (1986) The effectiveness and cost of home care, an information synthesis. *Health Services Research*, **20**, 851–80.

221. Pryor, G.A. and Williams, D.R.R. (1989) Rehabilitation after hip fractures. Home and hospital management compared. *The Journal of Bone and Joint Surgery*, **71**–B, 471–3.

222. Adler, M.W., Waller, J.J., Creese, A. and Thorne, S.C. (1978) Randomised controlled trial of early discharge for inguinal hernia and varicose veins. *Journal of Epidemiology and Community Health*, **32**, 136–42.

223. Aday, L.A., Wegener, R.M., Andersen, M.J. and Aitken, M.J. (1989) Home care for ventilator assisted children. *Health Affairs*, **14**, 137–47.

224. Welsh Health Planning Forum (1992) *Health and Social Care 2010*, Welsh Office, Cardiff.

225. Morris, P. (1992) Paediatric day case surgery. *British Journal of Anaesthesia*, **68**, 3–4.

226. Sadler, G.P., Richards, H., Watkins, G. and Foster, M.E. (1992) Day case paediatric surgery, the only choice. *Annals of the Royal College of Surgeons of England*, **74**, 130–3.

227. Drummond, M.F. and Yates, J.M. (1991) Clearing the cataract backlog in a (not so) developing country. *Eye*, **5**, 481–6.

228. Taylor, J., Goodman, M. and Luesley, D. (1993) Is home best? *Nursing Times*, **89**, 31–3.

229. Gamble, A.R., Bell, J.A., Ronan, J.E. *et al.* (1993) Use of tumour marker immunoreactivity to identify primary site of metastatic cancer. *British Medical Journal*, **306**, 295–7.

230. Dedman, P. (1993) Home treatment for acute psychiatric disorder. *British Medical Journal*, **306**, 1359–60.

231. Dean, C. and Gadd, E.M. (1990) Home treatment for acute psychiatric illness. *British Medical Journal*, **301**, 1021–3.

232. Stein, L.I. and Test, M.A. (1980) Alternative to mental hospital treatment. 1. Conceptual model, treatment program and clinical evaluation. *Archives of General Psychiatry*, **37**, 392–7.

233. Mulder, R. (1985) *Evaluation of the Harbinger Program 1982–1985*, Michigan Department of Mental Health, Lansing, MI.

234. Dean, C. and Gadd, E.M. (1990) Home treatment for acute psychiatric illness. *British Medical Journal*, **301**, 1021–3.

235. Muijen, M., Marks, I., Connolly, J., Audini, B. and McNamee, G. (1992) Home based care and standard hospital care for patients with severe mental illness, a randomised controlled trial. *British Medical Journal*, **304**, 749–54.

236. Burns, T., Raftery, J., Beadsmoore, A. *et al.* (1993) A controlled trial of home based

psychiatric services. II Treatment patterns and costs. *British Journal of Psychiatry*, **163**, 55–61.

237. Russell, I.T., Devlin, H.B., Fell, M. *et al.* (1977) Day case surgery for hernias and haemorrhoids, a clinical, social and economic evaluation. *The Lancet*, **1**, 844–7.

238. Audit Commission (1992) *A Short Cut to Better Services. Day Surgery in England and Wales*, HMSO, London.

239. Creditor, M.C. (1993) Hazards of hospitalization of the elderly. *Annals of Internal Medicine*, **118**, 219–23.

240. Chad, D.A. and Recht, L.D. (1991) Neuromuscular complications of systemic cancer. *Neurologic Clinics*, **9**, 901–18.

241. Potts, S., Feinglass, J., Lefevere, F. *et al.* (1993) A quality of care analysis of cascade iatrogenesis in frail elderly hospital patients. *Quality Review Bulletin*, **19**, 199–205.

242. Bomhof, J., Nieman, F.H. and Reerink, E. (1993) Registration of adverse patient occurrences in a university hospital, relations between adverse patient occurrences and characteristics of hospitalised patients. *Quality Assurance in Health Care*, **5**, 167–74.

243. Barbour, G.L. (1993) Usefulness of a discharge diagnosis of sepsis in detecting iatrogenic infection and quality of care problems. *American Journal of Medical Quality*, **8**, 2–5.

244. Lefevre, F., Feinglass, J., Potts, S. *et al.* (1992) Iatrogenic complications in high risk, elderly patients. *Archives of Internal Medicine*, **152**, 2074–80.

245. Ferraris, V.A. and Propp, M.E. (1992) Outcome in critical care patients, a multivariate study. *Critical Care Medicine*, **20**, 967–76.

246. Thompson, T.L. and Smith, T.C. (1991) Costumed figures may produce iatrogenic symptoms in delirious patients. *Psychosomatics*, **32**, 1–4.

247. Fraser, F.W. (1979) Evaluation of a Domiciliary Physiotherapy Service to the Elderly. Dissertation, The University of Aston.

248. Garraway, W.M., Akhtar, A.J., Hockey, L. and Prescott, R.J. (1980) Management of acute stroke in the elderly: Follow-up of a controlled trial. *British Medical Journal*, **281**, 827–9.

249. Research Unit of the Royal College of Physicians and the British Geriatrics Society (1992) *Standardised Assessment Scales for Elderly People*, Royal College of Physicians and the British Geriatrics Society, London.

250. Lorig, K., Feigenbaum, P., Regan, C. *et al.* (1986) A comparison of lay taught and professional taught arthritis self management courses. *The Journal of Rheumatology*, **13**, 763–7.

251. Zapka, J. and Mazur, R. (1977) Peer sex education training and evaluation. *American Journal of Public Health*, **67**, 450–4.

252. Cox, C.A. (1979) A pilot study, using the elderly as community health educators. *International Journal of Health Education*, **22**, 49–52.

253. Thompson, L.W., Gallagher, D. and Nies, G. (1983) Evaluation of the effectiveness of professionals and non-professionals as instructors of 'coping with depression' classes for elders. *The Gerontologist*, **23**, 390–6.

254. Perry, J.D. and Hullett, L.T. (1990) The role of home trainers in Kegel's exercise program for the treatment of incontinence. *Ostomy Wound Management*, **30**, 46–57.

255. Bandura, A., Blanchard, E. and Ritter, B. (1969) Relative efficiency of desensitization and modelling therapeutic approaches for inducing behavioural, affective and attitude changes. *Journal of Personal and Social Psychology*, **13**, 173–9.

256. Bandura, A., Jeffrey, R.W. and Wright, C.L. (1974) Efficacy of participant modelling as a function of response induction aids. *Journal of Abnormal Psychology*, **83** 56–64.

257. Cox, C.A. (1979) A pilot study, using the elderly as community health educators *International Journal of Health Education*, **22**, 49–52.

258. Bergner, M., Hudson, L.D., Conrad, D.A. *et al.* (1988) The cost and efficacy of home care for patients with chronic lung disease. *Medical Care*, **26**, 566–79.

259. Cherkasky, M. (1949) The Montefiore hospital home care program. *American Journal of Public Health*, **39**, 163–70.

260. US General Accounting Office (1982) *Report to the Chairman of the Committee on Labor and Human Resources*, US Senate GAO/IPE 83–1, Washington DC.

261. Stuck, A.E., Siu, A.L., Wieland, G.D. *et al.* (1993) Comprehensive geriatric assessment, a meta-analysis of controlled trials. *The Lancet*, **2**, 1032–6.

262. Fordham, R., Thompson, R., Holmes, J. and Hodkinson, C. (1986) A cost benefit study of geriatric orthopaedic management of patients with fractured neck of femur. Discussion paper 14 ed. University of York, Centre for Health Economics.

263. Gilchrist, W.J., Newman, R.J., Hamblen, D.L. and Williams, B.O. (1988) Prospective randomised study of an orthopaedic geriatric inpatient service. *British Medical Journal*, **297**, 1116–8.

264. Reid, J. and Kennie, D.C. (1989) Geriatric rehabilitative care after fractures of the proximal femur, one year follow up of a randomised controlled trial. *British Medical Journal*, **299**, 25–6.

265. Briggs, R.S.J. (1993) Orthogeriatric care and its effect on outcome. *Journal of the Royal Society of Medicine*, **86**, 560–2.

266. Tropman, J.E. (1987) Organisational excellence and the nursing home: a new perspective on quality of life. *Danish Medical Bulletin. Special Supplement Series*, No. 5, 2–6.

267. Department of Health (1990) *National Health Service and Community Care Act*, HMSO, London.

268. Laing, W. (1991) *Empowering the Elderly: Direct Consumer Funding of Care Services*, IEA Health and Welfare Unit, London.

269. Lewis, P.A., Dunn, R.B. and Vetter, N.J. (1994) NHS and community care act 1990 and discharges from hospital to private residential and nursing homes. *British Medical Journal*, **309**, 28–9.

270. Welsh Health Planning Forum (1989) *Local Strategies for Health: A New Approach to Strategic Planning*, Welsh Office, NHS Directorate, Cardiff.

271. NHS Wales (1994) *Caring for the Future*, Welsh Office, Cardiff.

272. WHO (1985) *Targets for Health for All. Target in Support of the European Regional Strategy for Health for All*, WHO Regional Office for Europe, Copenhagen.

273. Majeed, F.A., Chaturvedi, N., Reading, R. and Ben-Shlomo, Y. (1994) Monitoring and promoting equity in primary and secondary care. *British Medical Journal*, **308**, 1426–9.

274. Challis, L. and Henwood, M. (1994) Equity in community care. *British Medical Journal*, **308**, 1496–9.

275. Dixon, J., Dinwoodie, M., Hodson, D. *et al.* (1994) Distribution of NHS funds between fundholding and non-fundholding practices. *British Medical Journal*, **309**, 30–4.

276. Dimond, B. (1994) How far can you go? *Health Service Journal*, **104**, 24–5.

277. Grimley Evans, J. (1990) How are the elderly different?, in *Improving the Health of Older People*, (eds R.L. Kane, J. Grimley Evans and D. Macfadyen), Oxford University Press, Oxford.

278. Donaldson, L.J. and Jagger, G. (1983) Survival and functional capacity: three year follow-up of an elderly population in hospitals and homes. *Journal of Epidemiology and Community Health*, **37**, 85–9.

279. Bowling, A., Formby, J., Grant, K. and Ebrahim, S. (1991) A randomised controlled trial of nursing home and long stay geriatric ward care for elderly people. *Age and Ageing*, **20**, 316–24.

280. Challis, D., Darton, R., Johnson, L. *et al.* (1991) An evaluation of an alternative to long-stay hospital care for frail elderly patients. *Age and Ageing*, **20**, 236–44.

281. Atkinson, D.A., Bond, J. and Gregson, B.A. (1986) The dependency characteristics of older people in long-term institutional care, in *Dependency and Interdependency in Old Age, Theoretical perspectives and Policy Alternatives* (eds C. Phillipson, M. Bernard and P. Strang), Croom Helm, Beckenham, pp. 257–69.

282. Anon (1991) *Discontinuing Care. Report of a Survey of District Health Authority Plans for Continuing Care of Elderly People*, Age Concern, London.

283. Salvage, A.V., Jones, D.A. and Vetter, N.J. (1989) Opinions of people aged over 75 on private and local authority residential care. *Age and Ageing*, **18**, 380–6.

284. Donaldson, C. and Bond, J. (1989) *Evaluation of Continuing Care Accommodation for Elderly People. Volume 6. Views of Relatives and Volunteers*, Health Care Research Unit, University of Newcastle.

285. Donaldson, L. and Bond, D. (1991) Cost of continuing care facilities in the evaluation of experimental national health service nursing homes. *Age and Ageing*, **20**, 160–8.

286. OPCS Monitor (1992) *General Household Survey, Carers in 1990*, Vol. SS 92/2, OPCS, London.

287. Levin, E., Moriarty, J. and Gorbach, P. (1994) *Better for the Break*, HMSO, London.

288. Brody, E.M., Johnsen, P.T., Fulcomer, M.C. and Lang, A.M. (1983) Women's changing roles and help to elderly parents, attitudes of three generations of women. *Journal of Gerontology*, **38**, 597–607.

289. Equal Opportunities Commission (1980) *The Experience of Caring for Elderly and Handicapped Dependents*, Equal Opportunities Commission, Manchester.

290. Levin, E., Sinclair, I.A.C. and Gorbach, P. (1989) *Families, Services and Confusion in Old Age*, Gower, Aldershot.

291. Oberlander, T.F., Pless, I.B. and Dougherty, G.E. (1993) Advice seeking and appropriate use of a pediatric emergency department. *American Journal of Diseases of Children*, **147**, 863–7.

292. Tomlinson, P.S., Kirschbaum, M., Tomczyk, B. and Peterson, J. (1993) The relationship of child acuity, maternal responses, nurse attitudes and contextual factors in the bone marrow transplant unit. *American Journal of Critical Care*, **2**, 246–52.

293. Bradley, J.S. (1993) Pediatric considerations. *Hospital Practice*, **28**, Suppl 1, 28–32.

294. Deaves, D.M. (1993) An assessment of the value of health education in the prevention of childhood asthma. *Journal of Advanced Nursing*, **18**, 354–63.

295. Brook, U., Mendelberg, A. and Helm, M. (1993) Increasing parental knowledge of asthma decreases the hospitalisation of the child. *Journal of Asthma*, **30**, 45–9.

296. Fletcher, H.J., Ibrahim, S.A. and Speight, N. (1990) Survey of asthma deaths in the Northern Region, 1970–1985. *Archives of Disease in Childhood*, **65**, 163–7.

297. Taylor, M.R. and O'Connor, P. (1989) Resident parents and shorter hospital stay. *Archives of Disease in Childhood*, **64**, 274–6.

298. Sainsbury, C.P., Gray, O.P., Cleary, J. *et al.* (1986) Care by parents of their children in hospital. *Archives of Disease in Childhood*, **61**, 612–5.

299. Royal College of Surgeons of England (1985) *Guidelines for Day Case Surgery*, Royal College of Surgeons, London.

300. Johnson, C.D. and Jarrett, P.E.M. (1990) Admission to hospital after day case surgery. *Annals of the Royal College of Surgeons of England*, **72**, 225–8.

301. Rudkin, G.E., Osborne, G.A. and Doyle, C.E. (1993) Assessment and selection of patients for day surgery in a public hospital. *The Medical Journal of Australia*, **158**, 308–12.

302. Lowe, K.J., Gregory, D.A., Jefferey, R.I. and Easty, D.L. (1991) Patient perceptions and social impact. Preliminary results of the Bristol MRC study. *Eye*, **5**, 373–8.

303. Victor, C.R. and Vetter, N.J. (1988) Preparing the elderly for discharge from hospital, a neglected aspect of patient care? *Age and Ageing*, **17**, 155–63.

304. Jones, D. and Lester, C. (1994) Hospital care and discharge, patients' and carers' opinions. *Age and Ageing*, **23**, 91–6.

305. Pratt, C., Schmall, V. and Wright, S. (1985) Burden and coping strategies of caregivers to Alzheimer's patients. *Family Relations*, **34**, 27–33.

306. Stephens, M., Kinney, J. and Ogrocki, P. (1991) Stressors and wellbeing among caregivers to older people with dementia. The in-home versus nursing home experience. *The Gerontologist*, **31**, 217–20.

307. Bowers, B. (1988) Family perceptions of nursing home care, a grounded theory study of family work in a nursing home. *The Gerontologist*, **28**, 361–5.

308. Toseland, R. and Rossiter, C. (1989) Group interventions to support family caregivers. A review and analysis. *The Gerontologist*, **29**, 438–41.

309. Stephens, G.L., Walsh, R.A. and Baldwin, B.A. (1993) Family caregivers of institutionalized and noninstitutionalized elderly individuals. *Nursing Clinics of North America*, **28**, 349–62.

310. Falloon, I.R.H., McGill, C.W., Boyd, J.L. and Pederson, J. (1987) Family management in the prevention of morbidity of schizophrenia, social outcome of a two year longitudinal study. *Psychological Medicine*, **17**, 59–66.

311. Smith, J. and Birchwood, M. (1990) Relatives and patients as partners in the management of schizophrenia. *British Journal of Psychiatry*, **156**, 654–60.

312. Birchwood, M., Smith, J. and Cochrane, R. (1992) Specific and non specific effects of educational intervention for families living with schizophrenia. *British Journal of Psychiatry*, **160**, 806–14.

313. Salvage, A.V., Vetter, N.J. and Jones, D.A. (1988) Attitudes to hospital care among a community sample of people aged 75 and older. *Age and Ageing*, **17**, 270–4.

314. Vetter, N.J., Jones, D.A. and Victor, C.R. (1984) Effect of health visitors working with elderly patients in general practice: a randomised controlled trial. *British Medical Journal*, **288**, 369–72.

315. Vetter, N.J., Lewis, P.A. and Llewellyn, L. (1992) Supporting elderly dependent people at home. *British Medical Journal*, **304**, 1290–2.

316. Isaacs, B. (1971) Geriatric patients, Do their families care? *British Medical Journal*, **263**, 282–6.

317. Koopman Boyden, P.G. and Wells, L.F. (1979) The problems arising from supporting the elderly at home. *New Zealand Medical Journal*, **89**, 265–8.

318. Nissel, M. (1984) The family costs of looking after handicapped elderly relatives. *Ageing and Society*, **4**, 185–204.

319. Brody, E.M. (1981) Women in the middle; family help and older people. *The Gerontologist*, **21**, 471–81.

320. Jones, D.A. and Vetter, N.J. (1984) A survey of those who care for the elderly at home: their problems and their needs. *Social Science and Medicine*, **19**, 511–4.

321. Equal Opportunities Commission (1980) *The Experience of Caring for Elderly and Handicapped Dependants, Survey Report*, Equal Opportunities Commission, Manchester.

322. Allen, I. (1983) *Short Stay Residential Care for the Elderly*, Policy Studies Institute, London.

323. Vetter, N.J. (1992) How to assess the value of the geriatric day hospital, a problem in operational research. *European Journal of Gerontology*, **1**, 194–205.

324. Carter, J. (1981) *Day Services for Adults: Somewhere to Go*, Allen and Unwin, London.

325. Edwards, C., Sinclair, I. and Gorbach, P. (1980) Day centres for the elderly, variations in type, provision and user response. *British Journal of Social Work*, **10**, 419–30.

326. Crosbie, D., Vickery, A. and Sinclair, I. (1988) Schemes and social workers, issues of time, pressure and training. *Social Work Education*, **7**, 30–4.

327. Packwood, T. (1980) Supporting the family, a study of the organisation and implications of the hospital provision of holiday relief for families caring for dependants at home. *Social Science and Medicine*, **14a**, 613–20.

328. Allen, I. (1983) *Short Stay Residential Care for the Elderly*, Policy Studies Institute, London.

329. Dawson, J. (1987) Evaluation of a community based night sitter service, in *Research in the Nursing Care of Elderly People* (ed. P. Fielding), Wiley, Chichester.

330. Boldy, D. and Kuh, D. (1984) Short term care for the elderly in residential homes. *British Journal of Social Work*, **14**, 173–5.

331. Rai, G.S., Bielawska, C., Murphy, P.J. and Wright, G. (1986) Hazards for elderly people admitted for respite and social care. *British Medical Journal*, **292**, 240–1.

332. Thornton, P. and Moore, J. (1980) *Placement of Elderly People in Private Households*, Department of Social Policy and Administration Research Monograph, University of Leeds.

333. Wenger, C. (1984) *The Supportive Network: Coping with Old Age*, Allen and Unwin, London.

334. Barr, J.K., Johnson, K.W. and Warshaw, L.J. (1992) Supporting the elderly, workplace programs for employed caregivers. *The Millbank Quarterly*, **70**, 509–33.

335. Stone, R.I. and Short, P.F. (1990) The competing demands of employment and informal caregiving to disabled elders. *Medical Care*, **28**, 513–26.

336. Gibeau, J.L. and Anastas, J.N. (1988) *Breadwinners and Caregivers, Supporting Workers Who Care for Elderly Family Members*, National Association of Area Agencies on Aging, Washington DC.

337. Scharlach, A.E. and Boyd, S.L. (1989) Caregiving and employment, result of an employee survey. *The Gerontologist*, **29**, 382–7.

338. Anon (1991) *Health Care Benefits Survey 1990: Report 3. Flexible Benefits Programs*, Foster Higgins, Princeton, NJ.

339. Fortune Magazine and John Hancock Financial Services (1989) Corporate and employee response to caring for the elderly, a national survey of US companies and the workforce. *Fortune Magazine* (in-house publication).

340. Anon (1990) *Work and Family Benefits Provided by Major US Employers in 1990*, Hewitt Associates, Lincolnshire, Illinois.

341. US Department of Labor (1990) *Employee Benefits in Medium and Large Firms*, Bureau of Labor Statistic Bulletin 2363, Washington DC.

342. Worman, D. (1990) The forgotten carers. *Personnel Management*, **48**, 44–7.

343. Anon (1992) *What if They Hurt Themselves?* Counsel and Care, London.

344. Anon (1984) *Home Life: a Code of Practice for Residential Care*, Centre for Policy on Ageing, London.

345. Hirschfeld, M.J. and Fleishman, R. (1990) Nursing home care for the elderly, in *Improving the Health of Older People: a World View* (eds R.L. Kane, J. Grimley Evans, D. Macfadyen), Oxford University Press, Oxford, pp. 473–90.

346. Ham, C. (1992) *The New National Health Service. Organization and Management*, Radcliffe Medical Press, Oxford.

347. Russell, B., Anderton, J.L., Cormack, J.J.C. *et al.* (1983) Management of hypertension – a study of hospital outpatient practice. *Journal of the Royal College of General Practitioners*, 221–7.

348. Stocking, B. (1993) Implementing the findings of effective care in pregnancy and childbirth in the United Kingdom. *The Millbank Quarterly*, **71**, 497–521.

349. Lomas, J., Sisk, J.E. and Stocking, B. (1993) From evidence to practice in the United States, the United Kingdom and Canada. *The Millbank Quarterly*, **71**, 405–10.

350. Delamothe, T. (1993) Wanted, guidelines that doctors will follow. *British Medical Journal*, **307**, 218–9.

351. Farmer, A. (1993) Medical practice guidelines, lessons from the United States. *British Medical Journal*, **307**, 313–7.

352. Appleby, J., Smith, P., Ranade, W. *et al.* (1994) Monitoring managed competition, in *Evaluating the NHS Reforms*, (eds R. Robinson and J. Le Grand), King's Fund Institute, London, pp. 24–53.

353. Ray, S.G., Griffith, M.J., Jamieson, S. *et al.* (1992) Impact of the recommendations of the British pacing and electrophysiology group on pacemaker prescription and on the immediate costs of pacing in the Northern region. *British Heart Journal*, **68**, 531–4.

354. Axt-Adam, P., van der Wouden, J.C. and van der Does, E. (1993) Influencing behaviour of physicians ordering laboratory tests, a literature study. *Medical Care*, **31**, 784–94.

355. Manchester, D. (1993) Neuroleptics, learning disability and the community, some history and mystery. *British Medical Journal*, **307**, 184–7.

356. Werner, M. (1993) Can medical decisions be standardised? Should they be? *Clinical Chemistry*, **39**, 1361–8.

357. Moote, C. (1993) Techniques for post-op pain management in the adult. *Canadian Journal of Anesthesia*, **40**, R19–28.

358. Kemp, J.P. (1993) Approaches to asthma management. Realities and recommendations. *Archives of Internal Medicine*, **153**, 805–12.

359. Royal College of Radiologists' Working Party (1992) Influence of the Royal College of Radiologists' guidelines on hospital practice: a multicentre study. *British Medical Journal*, **304**, 740–3.

360. Pashkow, F.J. (1993) Issues in contemporary cardiac rehabilitation, a historical perspective. *Journal of the American College of Cardiology*, **21**, 822–34.
361. McWhirter, J.P. and Pennington, C.R. (1994) Incidence and recognition of malnutrition in hospital. *British Medical Journal*, **308**, 945–8.
362. Bistrian, B.R., Blackburn, G.L., Vitale, J. *et al.* (1976) Prevalence of malnutrition in general medical patients. *Journal of the American Medical Association*, **253**, 1567–70.
363. Hill, G.L., Pickford, J., Young, G.A. *et al.* (1977) Malnutrition in surgical patients, an unrecognised problem. *The Lancet*, **1**, 689–92.
364. Windsor, J.A. and Hill, G.L. (1988) Risk factors for post operative pneumonia, the importance of protein depletion. *Annals of Surgery*, **17**, 181–5.
365. Robinson, G., Goldstein, M. and Levine, G.M. (1987) Impact of nutritional status on DRG length of stay. *Journal of Parenteral and Enteral Nutrition*, **11**, 49–51.
366. Garrow, J. (1994) Starvation in hospital. *British Medical Journal*, **308**, 934–5.
367. Silagy, C. (1993) Developing a register of randomised controlled trials in primary care. *British Medical Journal*, **306**, 897–900.
368. Harris, A. (1993) Developing a research and development strategy for primary care. *British Medical Journal*, **306**, 189–92.
369. Hutchinson, A. and Fowler, P. (1992) Outcome measures for primary health care, what are the research priorities? *British Journal of General Practice*, **42**, 227–31.
370. Muijen, M., Marks, I., Connolly, J. *et al.* (1992) Home based care and standard hospital care for patients with severe mental illness, a randomised controlled trial. *British Medical Journal*, **304**, 749–54.
371. Melia, R.J., Morgan, M., Wolfe, C.D. and Swan, A.V. (1991) Consumers' views of the maternity services, implications for change and quality assurance. *Journal of Public Health Medicine*, **13**, 120–6.
372. Anon (1985) *Americans and their Doctors*, Louis Harris and Associates, New York.
373. Donabedian, A. (1966) Evaluating the quality of medical care. *Millbank Memorial Fund Quarterly*, **44**, 166–203.
374. Sisk, J.E., Dougherty, D.M., Ehrenhaft, P.M. *et al.* (1990) Assessing information for consumers on the quality of medical care. *Inquiry*, **27**, 263–72.
375. NHS Executive (1994) *Hospital and Ambulance Services Comparative Performance Guide 1993–1994*, The NHS Executive, London.
376. Harrison, A. and Bruscini, S. (eds) (1993) Concluding comment, in *Health Care UK 1992/93*, King's Fund Institute, London, pp. 97–8.
377. Turner, R. (1993) Big brother is looking after your health. *British Medical Journal*, **307**, 1623–4.
378. Graffy, J.P. and Williams, J. (1994) Purchasing for all, an alternative to fundholding. *British Medical Journal*, **308**, 391–4.
379. Tonks, A. (1994) Fundholders to take over all purchasing. *British Medical Journal*, **308**, 360–1.
380. Department of Health (1993) *Hospital doctors. Training for the future 'The Calman Report'*, HMSO, London.
381. Peters, T.J. and Waterman, R.H. (1982) *In Search of Excellence, Lessons from America's Best Run Companies*, Harper Collins, New York.
382. Pettigrew, A., Ferlie, E. and McKee, L. (1992) *Shaping Strategic Change, Making Change in Large Organisations: the Case of the National Health Service*, Sage, London.
383. Ham, C. and Hill, M. (1984) *The Policy Process in the Modern Capitalist State*, Wheatsheaf Books, Brighton.

384. Johnson, G. and Scholes, K. (1988) *Exploring Corporate Strategy*, 2nd edn, Prentice Hall, New York.

385. Turrill, T. (1986) *Change and innovation, a challenge for the NHS*. Institute of Health Services Management, London, IHSM Series 10.

386. Pascale, R. (1990) *Managing in the Edge*, Penguin Books, London.

387. Plant, R. (1987) *Managing Change and Making it Stick*, Fontana, London.

388. Appleby, J., Smith, P., Ranade, W. *et al.* (1994) Monitoring managed competition, in *Evaluating the NHS Reforms* (eds R. Robinson and J. Le Grand), King's Fund Institute, London, pp. 24–53.

389. Stocking, B. (1985) *Initiative and Inertia. Case Studies in the NHS*, Nuffield Provincial Hospitals Trust, London.

390. Revans, R.W. (1962) The hospital as a human system. *Physics in Medicine and Biology*, 7, 147–51.

391. Illiffe, S. and Haines, A. (1989) Developments in British General Practice. *Family Medicine*, 21, 169–76.

392. Neufeld, V.R., Bearpark, S. and Winterton, C. (1989) Optimal outcomes of clinical education, in *Clinical Education and the Doctor of Tomorrow* (eds B. Gastell and D.E. Rogers), New York Academy of Medicine, New York.

393. Medawar, C. (1984) *The Wrong Kind of Medicine*, Consumers Association, London.

394. Education Committee (1993) *Recommendations on Undergraduate Medical Training*, General Medical Council, London.

395. Pickering, G.W. (1968) *High Blood Pressure*, 2nd edn, Churchill, London.

396. Goldberg, D. (1991) Filters to care – a model, in *Indicators for Mental Health in the Population* (eds R. Jenkins and S. Griffiths), HMSO, London, pp. 30–7.

397. Rose, G. (1993) Mental disorders and the strategies of prevention. *Psychological Medicine*, 23, 553–5.

398. Rose, G. and Day, S. (1990) The population mean predicts the number of deviant individuals. *British Medical Journal*, 301, 1031–4.

399. Gurland, B., Copeland, J., Kuriansky, J. *et al.* (1983) *The Mind and Mood of Aging. Mental Health Problems of the Community Elderly in New York and London*, Haworth Press, New York.

400. Tudor Hart, J. (1985) The world turned upside down, proposals for community base undergraduate medical education. *Journal of the Royal College of General Practitioners*, 35, 63–8.

401. McManus, I.C. and Wakeford, R.E. (1989) A core medical curriculum. *British Medical Journal*, 302, 1051–2.

402. Spaulding, W.B. (1991) *Revitalizing Medical Education. McMaster Medical School*, Decker, Hamilton, Ontario, BC.

403. Forster, D.P., Drinkwater, C.K., Corradine, A. and Cowley, K. (1992) The family study, a model for integrating the individual and community perspective in medical education. *Medical Education*, 26, 110–5.

404. Kamien, M. (1990) Can first year medical students contribute to better care for patients with chronic disease? *Medical Education*, 24, 23–6.

405. Schmidt, H.G., Dauphinee, W.D. and Patel, V.L. (1987) Comparing the effects of problem based and conventional curricula in an international sample. *Journal of Medical Education*, 62, 305–15.

406. Friedman, C.P., DeBliek, R., Greer, D.S. *et al.* (1990) Charting the winds of change, evaluating innovative curricula. *Academic Medicine*, 65, 8–14.

407. Hamad, B. (1991) Community orientated medical education – what is it? *Medical Education*, **25**, 16–22.
408. Neufeld, V.R., Woodward, C.A. and MacLeod, S.M. (1989) The McMaster MD program, a case study of renewal in medical education. *Academic Medicine*, **23**, 423–32.
409. Welsh Health Planning Forum (1992) *Health and Social Care 2010*, Welsh Office, Cardiff.
410. National Association of Health Authorities and Trusts (1993) *Reinventing Healthcare: Towards a New Model*, NAHAT, Birmingham.
411. Department of Health (1991) *The Health of the Nation*, HMSO, London.
412. West, M. and Anderson, N. (1993) Fire fighting. *Health Service Journal*, **103**, 20–4.
413. Poulton, B.C. and West, M.A. (1993) Effective multidisciplinary teamwork in primary health care. *Journal of Advanced Nursing*, **18**, 918–25.
414. Braun, P., Kochansky, G., Shapiro, R. *et al.* (1981) Overview, deinstitutionalization of psychiatric patients, a critical review of outcome studies. *American Journal of Psychiatry*, **138**, 736–49.
415. Tansella, M. (1986) Community psychiatry without mental hospitals – the Italian experience, a review. *Journal of the Royal Society of Medicine*, **79**, 664–9.
416. World Health Organization (1978) *Primary Health Care*, Alma Ata. Health for All Series No. 1, World Health Organization, Geneva.
417. Macagba, R. (1985) *Hospitals and Primary Health Care*, International Hospital Federation, London.
418. Mahler, H. (1975) Health – a demystification of medical technology. *The Lancet*, **2**, 829–33.
419. Klein, R. (1991) On the Oregon trail. *British Medical Journal*, **302**, 1–2.
420. Roberts, F. (1952) *The Cost of Health*, Turnstile Press, London.
421. Miller, H. (1973) *Medicine and Society*, Oxford University Press, London.

Index